AF902890

Total-Body PET/CT

Hongcheng Shi • Guobing Liu
Yiqiu Zhang • Hui Tan • Pengcheng Hu
Editors

Total-Body PET/CT

Prospective Clinical Applications

SSTP

Springer

Editors
Hongcheng Shi
Nuclear Medicine
Zhongshan Hospital
Shanghai, China

Guobing Liu
Nuclear Medicine
Zhongshan Hospital
Shanghai, China

Yiqiu Zhang
Nuclear Medicine
Zhongshan Hospital
Shanghai, China

Hui Tan
Nuclear Medicine
Zhongshan Hospital
Shanghai, China

Pengcheng Hu
Nuclear Medicine
Zhongshan Hospital
Shanghai, China

ISBN 978-981-97-5064-1 ISBN 978-981-97-5065-8 (eBook)
https://doi.org/10.1007/978-981-97-5065-8

© Shanghai Scientific and Technical Publishers 2024

Jointly published with Shanghai Scientific and Technical Publishers
The print edition is not for sale in China (Mainland). Customers from China (Mainland) please order the print book from: Shanghai Scientific and Technical Publishers.
This work is subject to copyright. All rights are solely and exclusively licensed by the Publisher, whether the whole or part of the material is concerned, specifically the rights of reprinting, reuse of illustrations, recitation, broadcasting, reproduction on microfilms or in any other physical way, and transmission or information storage and retrieval, electronic adaptation, computer software, or by similar or dissimilar methodology now known or hereafter developed.
The use of general descriptive names, registered names, trademarks, service marks, etc. in this publication does not imply, even in the absence of a specific statement, that such names are exempt from the relevant protective laws and regulations and therefore free for general use.
The publishers, the authors, and the editors are safe to assume that the advice and information in this book are believed to be true and accurate at the date of publication. Neither the publishers nor the authors or the editors give a warranty, express or implied, with respect to the material contained herein or for any errors or omissions that may have been made. The publishers remain neutral with regard to jurisdictional claims in published maps and institutional affiliations.

This Springer imprint is published by the registered company Springer Nature Singapore Pte Ltd.
The registered company address is: 152 Beach Road, #21-01/04 Gateway East, Singapore 189721, Singapore

If disposing of this product, please recycle the paper.

Foreword

In April 2019, the world's first total-body PET/CT with a 194-cm axial field of view, developed by Shanghai United Imaging Healthcare Co., Ltd., was installed in Zhongshan Hospital, Fudan University. Professor Hongcheng Shi and his team from the Department of Nuclear Medicine, leveraging the comprehensive strength of Zhongshan Hospital, embarked on a series of clinical application exploration researches, beginning with the resolution of difficult and key problems in medical work. This research included a model-based experimental study, which verified the excellent performance of total-body PET/CT compared with conventional PET/CT. On this basis, clinical trials were conducted to assess the feasibility and diagnostic efficacy of total-body PET/CT, which is able to complete the examination in 30 s and obtain high-quality diagnostic results in 2 min. For the first time, dynamic images acquired via total-body PET/CT were used to display the whole process of the distribution of radiotracer ^{18}F-FDG in the body, thus introducing the concept of visual pharmacodynamics and pharmacokinetics, laying the groundwork for further in-depth research. Besides, the clinical application value of parametric imaging was explored, and the gain value of the time–activity curve in the differential diagnosis of the liver tumor was determined. Furthermore, it was confirmed that the imaging of ^{18}F-FDG at one-tenth ultra-low dose was comparable to conventional PET/CT, except for the peak value. The feasibility of total-body PET/CT imaging with a one-tenth dose was also confirmed, and the parameter settings of one-tenth dose and half-dose imaging technology were further optimized. Finally, operational specifications of total-body PET/CT were established, providing a solid foundation for the popularization and standardized clinical application of this innovative equipment.

For over 3 years, Professor Hongcheng Shi's team has been exploring the implications of total-body PET/CT with innovative academic perspectives while also furthering the production of high-quality scientific research results through collaborative efforts between the team and medical enterprises, thus pooling the collective wisdom of many and forming an excellent team. Notably, their pioneering research has enabled more patients, who were previously unable to accept PET/CT examination, to benefit from the advanced medical equipment through rapid total-body PET/CT scanning, ultra-low dose imaging, and other methods, and this approach has become the preferred choice in clinical imaging examinations.

The clinical exploration application of the world's first total-body PET/CT at Zhongshan Hospital reflects the comprehensive and in-depth collaboration between Zhongshan Hospital and United Imaging Healthcare, which fully embraces the development concept of Zhongshan Hospital of "innovation, cooperation, wisdom, quality and efficiency." In this process, the team of the Department of Nuclear Medicine of Zhongshan Hospital has been strengthened, and the level of discipline has been significantly improved. It is hoped that in the subsequent clinical exploration, Professor Hongcheng Shi's team can confer this advanced medical imaging equipment with greater practical value and provide patients with high-quality and innovative results.

Jia Fan

Academician of Chinese Academy
of Sciences, Zhongshan Hospital,
Fudan University
Shanghai, China
27 March 2023

Preface

This book is based on systematic clinical exploratory studies of more than 4 years on the world's first total-body positron emission tomography–computed tomography (PET/CT) with an axial field of view of 194 cm. This book summarizes the "Zhongshan Experience" gained from these studies.

This book comprises ten chapters that are both self-contained and interrelated. It begins with a concise introduction to the physical properties and potential clinical advantages of total-body PET/CT, accompanied by an exploration of a variety of clinical applications to transform these potential benefits into effective strategies to address clinical issues. Firstly, comparative studies between total-body PET/CT and conventional digital PET/CT have demonstrated the feasibility and diagnostic efficacy of fast scans. Secondly, the unique value and potential benefits of total-body dynamic acquisition in pharmacokinetic studies have been determined, along with the value of parameter imaging and time–activity curves derived from dynamic acquisition images for tumor diagnosis. Furthermore, the feasibility and optimization of imaging settings for half-dose and ultra-low-dose (1/10) total-body PET/CT scans are described. Moreover, new technologies, such as gating technology and ultra-low-dose CT, are introduced, which are currently being explored and improved. Finally, this book discusses the particulars of the expert consensus on ^{18}F-FDG total-body PET/CT in tumor imaging and presents our preliminary experience of the workflow of total-body PET/CT examinations in various application scenarios.

Shanghai, China
27 March 2023

Hongcheng Shi

Introduction

Total-body (TB) positron emission tomography–computed tomography (PET/CT), with a 194-cm axial field of view (AFOV), is capable of providing comprehensive imaging from the vertex to the toes in a single-bed scan, which is in marked contrast to conventional PET/CT with a 15–30 cm AFOV, which requires multiple bed scans to generate whole-body imaging, extending from the vertex to the mid-thigh. TB PET/CT has the ability to "capture" the lesions over the entire body, but more importantly, because of its extended AFOV, the count rate of TB PET/CT is approximately 40 times that of conventional PET/CT with a 20-cm AFOV. This heightened sensitivity has numerous implications and significantly enhances its clinical service capabilities.

In April 2019, Zhongshan Hospital, affiliated to Fudan University, became the first global user of the TB PET/CT (uEXPLORER, United Imaging, Shanghai, China), thus inaugurating a new era of total-body PET/CT clinical application. By the end of 2022, after more than 3 years of clinical application exploration, research on medical imaging data of over 20,000 cases (including 1764 dynamic acquisitions) has been published in over 30 academic articles in influential medical imaging journals in China and abroad, and our staff have been invited to present, exchange, and promote our experience at numerous local and international academic conferences. This has gained widespread attention and high recognition from the industry.

The proliferation of the TB PET/CT imaging tool has been noteworthy in the field of nuclear medicine, with its use becoming increasingly commonplace in clinical settings. Despite this, there remains a lack of authoritative references and professional literature in this area. This book serves as a compendium of the stage-by-stage findings of the editorial team, which are presented in terms of the clinical utility of TB PET/CT, strategies for addressing clinical issues, and the research methods employed during the process of clinical application exploration. As a single-center, stage-by-stage study, it has both strengths and weaknesses, which are presented to the readers here in the hope that it might serve as a beacon for this field's ongoing journey of discovery.

Department of Nuclear Medicine
Zhongshan Hospital, Fudan University
Shanghai, China

Hongcheng Shi

Acknowledgment

Dedicated to the 66th anniversary of the establishment of the Nuclear Medicine Department at Zhongshan Hospital, Fudan University.

Contents

Editors and Contributors

Editors

Hongcheng Shi Department of Nuclear Medicine, Zhongshan Hospital, Fudan University, Shanghai, China

Guobing Liu Department of Nuclear Medicine, Zhongshan Hospital, Fudan University, Shanghai, China

Yiqiu Zhang Department of Nuclear Medicine, Zhongshan Hospital, Fudan University, Shanghai, China

Hui Tan Department of Nuclear Medicine, Zhongshan Hospital, Fudan University, Shanghai, China

Pengcheng Hu Department of Nuclear Medicine, Zhongshan Hospital, Fudan University, Shanghai, China

Contributors

Dilibire Adili Department of Nuclear Medicine, Zhongshan Hospital, Fudan University, Shanghai, China

Danjie Cai Department of Nuclear Medicine, Zhongshan Hospital, Fudan University, Shanghai, China

Shuguang Chen Department of Nuclear Medicine, Zhongshan Hospital, Fudan University, Shanghai, China

Xueqi Chen Department of Nuclear Medicine, Zhongshan Hospital, Fudan University, Shanghai, China

Huaping Gao Department of Nuclear Medicine, Zhongshan Hospital, Fudan University, Shanghai, China

Yushen Gu Department of Nuclear Medicine, Zhongshan Hospital, Fudan University, Shanghai, China

Yibo He Department of Nuclear Medicine, Zhongshan Hospital, Fudan University, Shanghai, China

Yan Hu Department of Nuclear Medicine, Zhongshan Hospital, Fudan University, Shanghai, China

Yu Lin Department of Nuclear Medicine, Zhongshan Hospital, Fudan University, Shanghai, China

Jing Lv Department of Nuclear Medicine, Zhongshan Hospital, Fudan University, Shanghai, China

Chi Qi Department of Nuclear Medicine, Zhongshan Hospital, Fudan University, Shanghai, China

Xiuli Sui Department of Nuclear Medicine, Zhongshan Hospital, Fudan University, Shanghai, China

Ha Wu Department of Nuclear Medicine, Zhongshan Hospital, Fudan University, Shanghai, China

Jie Xiao Department of Nuclear Medicine, Zhongshan Hospital, Fudan University, Shanghai, China

Runjun Yang Department of Nuclear Medicine, Zhongshan Hospital, Fudan University, Shanghai, China

Haojun Yu Department of Nuclear Medicine, Zhongshan Hospital, Fudan University, Shanghai, China

Zhe Zheng Department of Nuclear Medicine, Zhongshan Hospital, Fudan University, Shanghai, China

Development, Characteristics, and Clinical Application of Total-Body PET/CT

1

Jing Lv, Danjie Cai, Guobing Liu, Jie Xiao, Yu Lin, Hui Tan, Yibo He, and Hongcheng Shi

In April 2019, the world's first total-body positron emission tomography computed tomography (TB PET/CT) with a 194-cm axial field of view (AFOV), the uEXPLORER, was installed at Zhongshan Hospital, affiliated to Fudan University, ushering in a new era of the clinical application of TB PET/CT.

1.1 A Brief History of PET/CT Development

In 1974, positron emission tomography (PET) (PETT III) was launched commercially. In 1998, David Townsend's team first used PET/CT for patient examination. In the same year, the USA Food and Drug Administration (FDA) approved ^{18}F-fluorodeoxyglucose (FDG) PET for cancer patient examination. The commercial operation of PET/CT began in 2000. With technological advances, PET/CT imaging equipment has been continuously improved and upgraded in terms of both hardware and software performance. For example, PET detectors have evolved from early sodium iodide crystals to bismuth germanite (BGO), then to lutetium oxyorthosilicate (LSO) and lutetium yttrium oxyorthosilicate (LYSO) [1], and eventually introducing the time-of-flight technology [2]; image reconstruction has progressed from the initial filtered back projection method to the ordered subset expectation maximization method. Meanwhile, CT in PET/CT has advanced from 1- or 2-detector-row scanners in the early stages to 64- or 128-detector-row scanners today. With the overall improvement of PET/CT performance and the deepening of its clinical application, its scope of application has continued to expand, and its role is increasingly being recognized. After more than two decades of development and improvement, PET/CT has become an advanced nuclear medicine molecular imaging technology and is the only imaging technology that is capable of displaying molecular metabolism, and receptor and neurotransmitter activity in vivo. However, there remain many challenges in the use of high-quality PET/CT images to capture tracer distribution information, detect early lesions more sensitively, and to evaluate dynamic changes of the lesions in the early stages.

The quality of PET/CT images is markedly impacted by multiple factors, such as the injection dose of radiotracers, the signal-to-noise ratio (SNR), imaging time, and equipment resolution. Currently, the AFOV of commercial conventional PET/CT is approximately 15–30 cm, and each bed scan can only cover around one-eighth of the body. The received signal is only around 1% of the number of photons emitted from the human body, which limits the detection efficiency and sensitivity of the system. Long axial field of view

J. Lv · D. Cai · G. Liu · J. Xiao · Y. Lin · H. Tan
Y. He · H. Shi (✉)
Department of Nuclear Medicine, Zhongshan Hospital, Fudan University, Shanghai, China
e-mail: shi.hongcheng@zs-hospital.sh.cn

© Shanghai Scientific and Technical Publishers 2024

H. Shi et al. (eds.), *Total-Body PET/CT*, https://doi.org/10.1007/978-981-97-5065-8_1

(LAFOV) PET/CT represents a breakthrough to overcome these impediments.

The concept of LAFOV PET/CT was initially proposed by Terry Jones in the early 1990s [3]. In June 2004, Japanese scholars introduced a PET/CT with a 68.5 cm AFOV (Hamamatsu SHR-92000) [4]; however, it was not implemented clinically. In 2018, the University of California, Davis and United Imaging Healthcare developed uEXPLORER, a TB PET/CT with a 194 cm LAFOV, which was subsequently established. The team from the Department of Nuclear Medicine of Zhongshan Hospital collaborated with the research and development team of uEXPLORER in the preclinical exploratory research of the equipment (Fig. 1.1). In January 2019, uEXPLORER obtained USA FDA approval, and in April 2019, the world's first LAFOV PET/CT (uEXPLORER) was installed in Zhongshan Hospital (Fig. 1.2) and began clinical validation [5, 6]. In December 2019, it received market authorization from the National Medical Products Administration (China).

In 2020, Biograph Vision Quadra PET/CT [7], developed by Siemens, with a 106 cm AFOV, was implemented clinically. The PennPET EXPLORER, a LAFOV PET/CT jointly developed by Philips and the University of Pennsylvania, is still in the research and development phase. Table 1.1 outlines the key parameters of the three LAFOV PET/CT scanners.

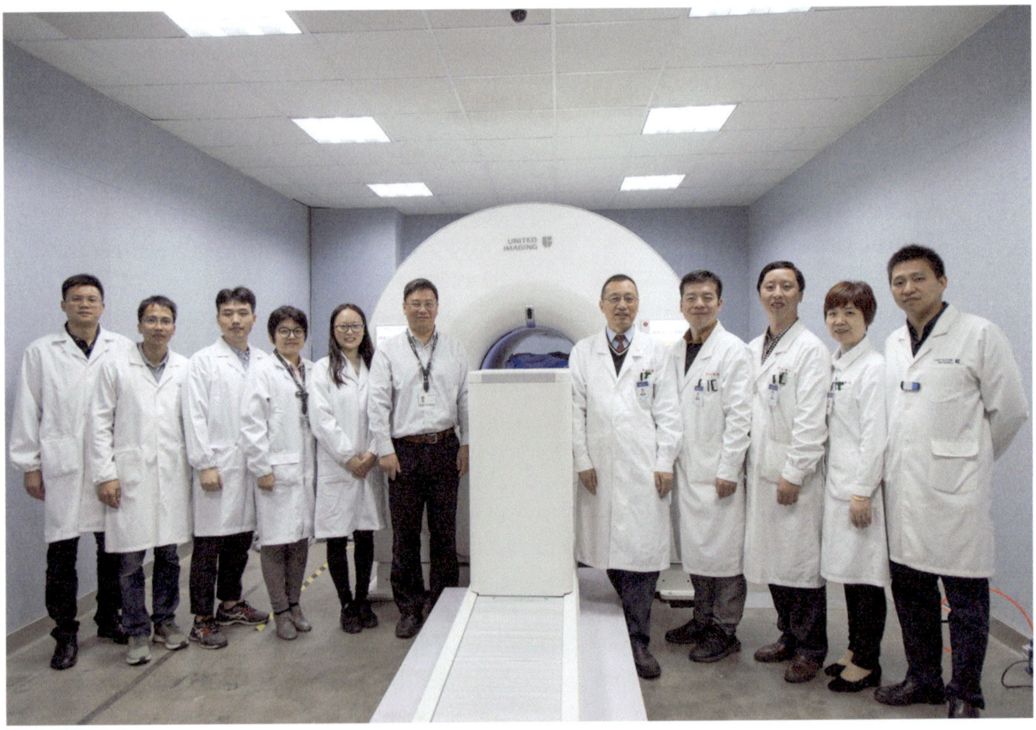

Fig. 1.1 The team from the Department of Nuclear Medicine of Zhongshan Hospital and the research and development team of uEXPLORER at the production site. In November 2018, the team from the Department of Nuclear Medicine of Zhongshan Hospital visited the production site of United Imaging Healthcare and discussed the potential clinical application of total-body PET/CT and its verification plan with the research and development team of uEXPLORER

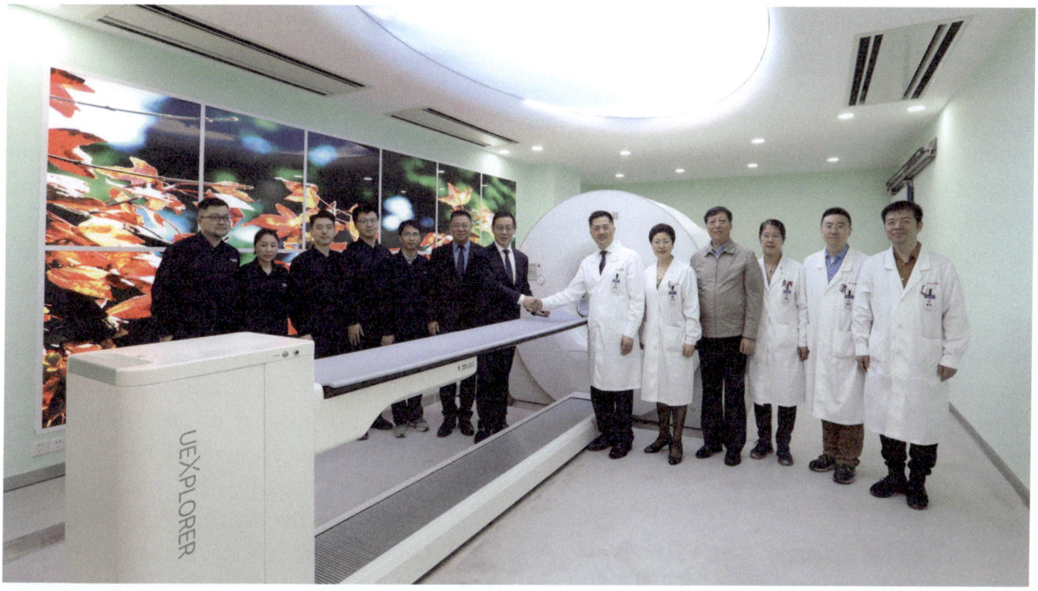

Fig. 1.2 Academician Jia Fan and Dr. Min Xue jointly launched the clinical application of uEXPLORER. In April 2019, the Chinese Academy of Science academician, Jia Fan (sixth from left), who is also the president of Zhongshan Hospital, affiliated to Fudan University, and the president of United Imaging Healthcare Co., Ltd., Min Xue (seventh from right) jointly launched the world's first total-body PET/CT (uEXPLORER) for clinical application in Zhongshan Hospital

Table 1.1 The key parameters of three LAFOV PET/CT scanners [8]

PET/CT	uEXPLORER	PennPET Explorer	Biograph Vision Quadra
Crystal	LYSO	LYSO	LSO
Crystal size (mm^3)	2.76 × 2.76 × 18.1	3.86 × 3.86 × 19	3.2 × 3.2 × 20
Inner diameter of the detector (cm)	68.6	70	78
Axial length (cm)	194.8	140	106
Energy resolution (%)	11.7	12	10.7
TOF resolution (ps)	430	250	228
Sensitivity kcps/MBq	174	55	174
Spatial resolution (mm)	2.9	4.0	3.3
Scattering fraction (%)	35.8	32	36

LYSO lutetium yttrium oxyorthosilicate, *LSO* lutetium oxyorthosilicate, *TOF* time-of-flight

1.2 Features and Potential Advantages of the uEXPLORER TB PET/CT

1.2.1 Physical Characteristics of TB PET/CT

The AFOV of uEXPLORER TB PET/CT is 194 cm, with a transverse field of view of 68.6 cm. Theoretically, the utilization of time-of-flight technology in a PET/CT with an AFOV of 194 cm yields a detection efficiency that is 40 times higher than that of a conventional PET/CT with an AFOV of 22 cm. Moreover, the uEXPLORER TB PET/CT can acquire a comprehensive image from head to toe in a single-bed position, which is a significant advantage over conventional PET/CT, which necessitates multiple bed positions to generate a stitched "whole-body" image from the head to the mid-thigh.

1.2.2 Potential Applications of TB PET/CT

The SNR is a key indicator for evaluating the quality of PET/CT images. SNR $\approx k\sqrt{S*A*T}$, where k is a constant, S represents the sensitivity, A represents the activity of the radiopharmaceutical, and T represents the acquisition time. The ultra-high sensitivity of uEXPLORER theoretically lays the foundation for improved image quality, shorter acquisition time, lower administered activity, the ability to acquire PET images at longer delayed time points, and the capacity to engage in pharmacokinetic parameter research.

1.3 Exploration of the Clinical Application of TB PET/CT

TB PET/CT (uEXPLORER) has an AFOV of 194 cm, providing an inherent advantage of single-bed, high-efficiency acquisition of total-body images from head to toe. This is in contrast to conventional PET/CT, which acquires "stitched" whole-body images from the head to the mid-thigh through partial overlap between multiple beds. The increased sensitivity conferred by the LAFOV further enhances the ability of TB PET/CT to detect smaller or low conspicuousness lesions (Fig. 1.3).

To effectively address the current clinical challenges in nuclear medicine using the advantages of TB PET/CT, the team from the Department of Nuclear Medicine at Zhongshan Hospital conducted a series of exploratory studies. They summarized the clinical advantages of uEXPLORER TB PET/CT and corresponding operational standards (Fig. 1.4).

1.3.1 Exploratory Research on Rapid Scanning

Based on a phantom and a clinical perspective study, the feasibility of uEXPLORER TB PET/CT fast scan was explored, and the parameters and acquisition conditions for a fast scan were established without compromising the image quality when compared with conventional PET/CT.

1.3.2 Exploratory Research on Pharmacokinetic Visualization

Traditional pharmacokinetic studies often focus solely on changes in blood drug concentrations, lacking information on drug distribution in various tissues and organs. To obtain the relevant information for a period of time after drug administration, precise pharmacological evaluation is required. The clinical application of TB PET has laid the foundation for visualizing pharmacokinetic studies and the use of uEXPLORER TB PET/CT in dynamic imaging of healthy volunteers has demonstrated, for the first time, the real-time imaging of the dynamic distribution of ^{18}F-FDG in the human body. This study has also revealed the dynamic distribution process of ^{18}F-FDG in different tissues and organs of the human body using semi-quantitative parameters.

1.3.3 Exploratory Research on Low-Dose Scanning

1.3.3.1 Half-Dose and Ultra-Low-Dose ^{18}F-FDG Activity

The uEXPLORER TB PET/CT was used to evaluate the dynamic distribution of radiotracers in healthy volunteers. The study found that, aside from differences in peak values, the distribution of ^{18}F-FDG in the human body was consistent between full dose (3.7 MBq/kg) and ultra-low dose (0.37 MBq/kg) ^{18}F-FDG PET imaging. This provides supportive evidence for the clinical application of ultra-low-dose (0.37 MBq/kg) ^{18}F-FDG TB PET imaging. Subsequently, a clinical study was conducted on a group of patients who underwent half-dose (1.75 MBq/kg) and ultra-low-dose (0.37 MBq/kg) ^{18}F-FDG TB PET imaging. The study found no significant difference in the distribution of half-dose and ultra-low-dose ^{18}F-FDG in the bodies of the patients, and the appropriate acquisition time did not affect the detection efficiency of lesions. This further confirmed the feasibility of using low and ultra-low-dose radiotracer in clinical applications. Finally, the study explored and established the acquisi-

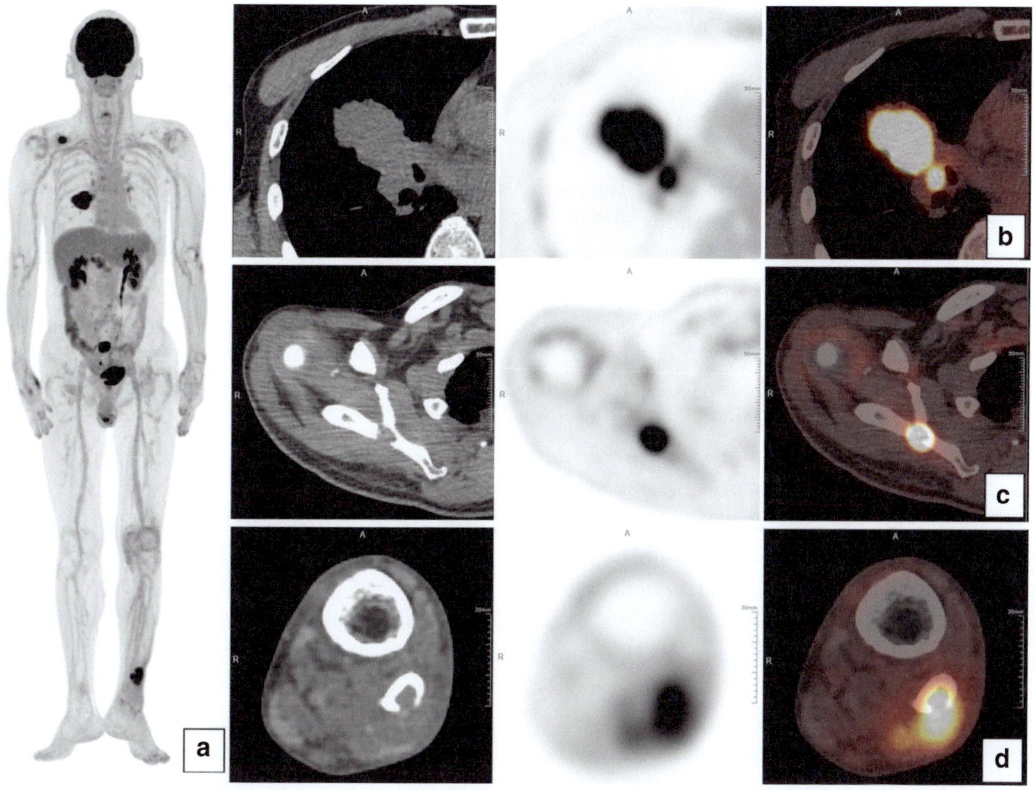

Fig. 1.3 A patient with central lung cancer in the right lung with metastases on the right scapula and left fibula. Maximum intensity projection (MIP) image of a 65-year-old male patient revealed abnormal radiotracer uptake in the right perihilar region of the lung, right scapula, and distal left fibula (**a**). The corresponding transaxial images demonstrate a focal increase in glucose metabolism adjacent to the right middle lobe bronchus (**b**), which protruded into the bronchial lumen, accompanied by an increase in glucose metabolism in the distal lung. Focal lytic bone destruction with an associated soft tissue mass is present in the right scapula (**c**) and the distal left fibula (**d**)

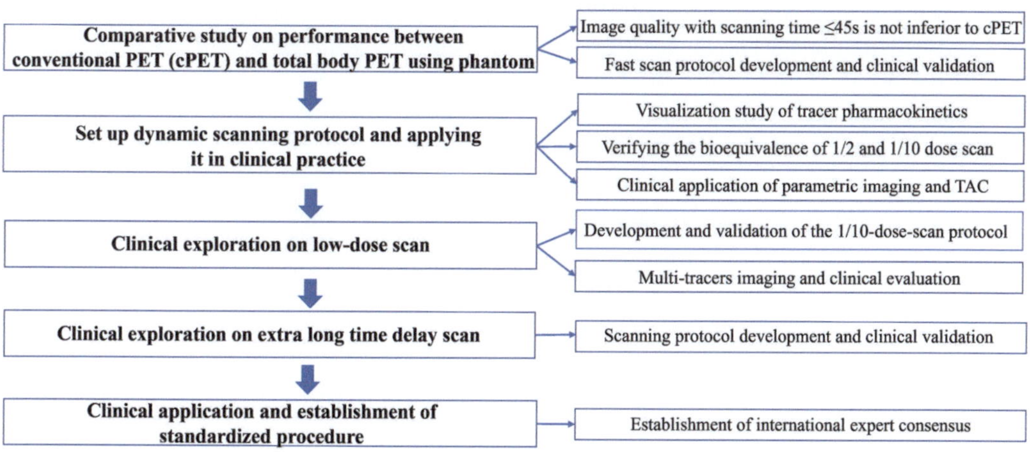

Fig. 1.4 Clinical application of the roadmap of TB PET/CT summarized by the nuclear medicine team of Zhongshan Hospital

tion parameters for half-dose and ultra-low-dose ^{18}F-FDG TB PET/CT imaging.

1.3.3.2 Personalized Injection Dose

Our team designed a cohort study to determine the efficacy of a personalized tracer injection dose based on the body mass index (BMI) of the patient to ensure PET image quality, where all included patients had similar pre-imaging conditions, such as fasting blood glucose levels <6.1 mmol/L [9]. The first cohort comprised 78 patients with cancer (59.7 ± 13.7 years old) who underwent full-dose ^{18}F-FDG TB PET/CT examination, and the obtained data were used to develop the dose regimen. Linear and non-linear methods were used to fit SNRnorm (normalized liver signal-to-noise ratio), which represents image quality, with patient-related parameters. The results showed that the linear fitting between SNRnorm and BMI demonstrated the best goodness of fit. Consequently, a recommended BMI-based injection dose regimen was derived: injection dose = 39.2 × MBq/(−0.03 × BMI + 1.49)^2. To further validate this BMI-based injection dose regimen, a second cohort of 38 patients with cancer was included. Personalized ^{18}F-FDG injection doses were calculated based on the injection dose formula, and TB PET/CT examination was performed using the personalized injection dose. The result for the second cohort indicated that the liver SNR (SNRL) images no longer decreased with increasing BMI, thus achieving homogeneous image quality. There was no statistically significant difference in the SNRL values of image quality between different BMI groups in the validation group ($p > 0.05$). In addition, compared with those in the first cohort using the conventional imaging agent dose model, the injection doses for the four different BMI groups in the second cohort were reduced by 75.6 ± 2.9%, 72.1 ± 4.0%, 67.1 ± 4.4%, and 64.8 ± 3.5%, respectively. This result suggested that the linear dose regimen based on BMI proposed in this study could achieve homogeneous image quality for patients with different BMIs, while the imaging agent dose given was lower than the recommended dose in the current guidelines. A typical case is shown in Fig. 1.5.

1.3.4 Application of Multi-Tracer Low-Dose Imaging

The application of multi-tracer low-dose imaging can provide complementary biological information between different tracers, thereby enhancing the efficacy of disease diagnosis or evaluation. However, the mutual interference of the radionuclides used in different tracers is a major impediment to the concurrent utilization of multiple tracers [10]. The use of low or ultra-low-dose multi-tracer TB PET/CT imaging on different days is a straightforward and convenient approach; however, it is time-consuming and not highly practicable. The same-day method can reduce the patient's multiple back-and-forth trips and effectively minimize time costs; however, it requires optimization of more reasonable and applicable imaging parameters to achieve a multi-tracer joint imaging method that is both expeditious and interpretable. Our team's related research is still ongoing.

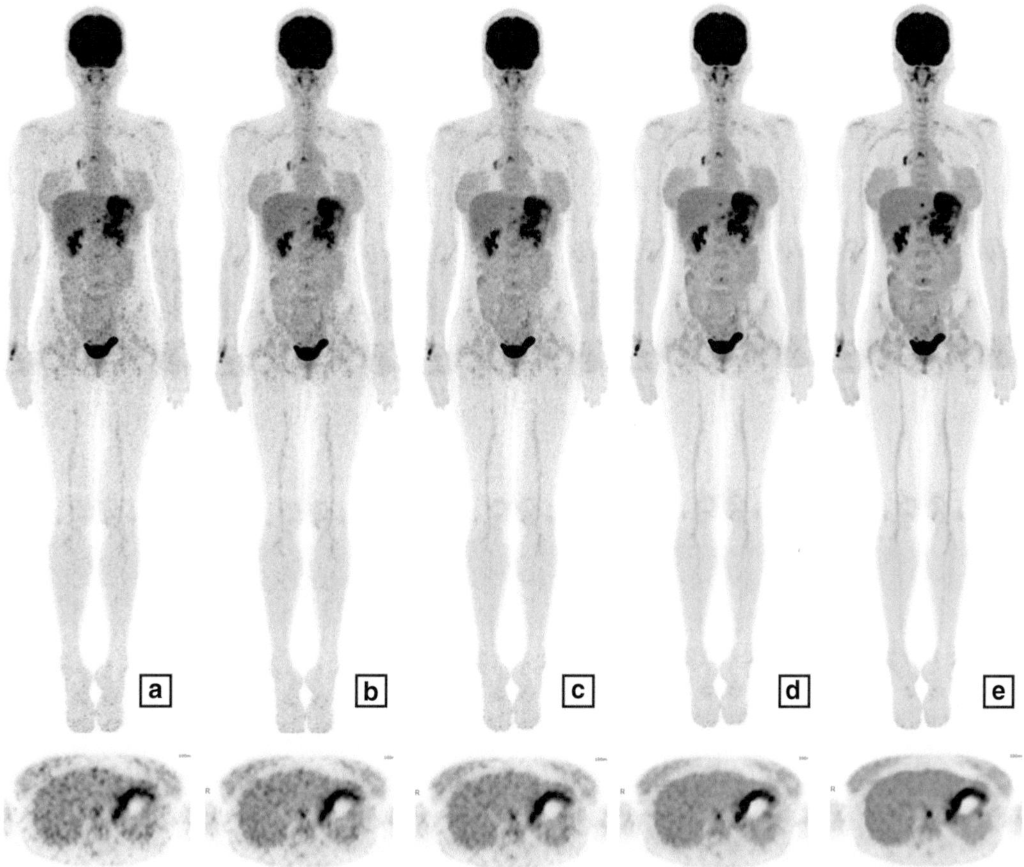

Fig. 1.5 Personalized injection dose TB PET/CT images with different acquisition times. A 32-year-old female of 171.1 cm in height and 51.7 kg in weight, and BMI of 17.7 kg/m^2, was given an injection of 40.7 MBq of ^{18}F-FDG, which was approximately 78.8% lower than the recommended dose of 191.3 MBq according to the personalized injection protocol. Images (**a**–**e**) represent images reconstructed for 30s, 45s, 60s, 120s and 300s, respectively. The image quality obtained with a scan time of 60 s was satisfactory for clinical diagnostic purposes

1.4 Current Achievements of the Exploratory Clinical Application of TB PET/CT

From April 2019 to December 2022, the Department of Nuclear Medicine at Zhongshan Hospital performed over 20,000 examinations using uEXPLORER PET/CT, including 1764 dynamic acquisitions encompassing a variety of tracers and different doses of the same tracer. Through a series of exploratory clinical studies, based on abundant detailed clinical evidence, significant progress has been made, clearly demonstrating the clinical application advantages of uEXPLORER TB PET/CT, including fast scanning, half or ultra-low-dose scanning, and dynamic scanning. Meanwhile, we have established the corresponding operational standards based on the clinical advantages of TB PET/CT, thereby enhancing the clinical service capacity of PET.

1.4.1 The Leap from Theoretical Inference to Clinical Application

Our team's exploratory research has established a personalized uEXPLORER TB PET/CT acquisition protocol, which has been published as an international expert consensus [11]. This protocol recommends an injection dose of 3.7 MBq/kg for ^{18}F-FDG in adults for a routine PET/CT examination with an AFOV of 15–30 cm, with an acquisition time of 2–3 min/bed and an average examination time of 15–30 min per person. The available options include fast scans for ^{18}F-FDG imaging with an injection dose according to guideline recommendations (3.7 MBq/kg), with standard acquisition times of 0.5–2 min and fast acquisition times of 0.51 min; half-dose (1.75 MBq/kg) ^{18}F-FDG imaging with standard acquisition times of 3–5 min and fast acquisition times of 2–4 min; and ultra-low-dose (0.37 MBq/kg) ^{18}F-FDG imaging with standard acquisition times of 7–15 min and fast acquisition times of 6–8 min. Delayed imaging and dynamic acquisition can be used to further enhance the sensitivity to detect specific lesions and to provide more detailed information on the lesions, respectively.

1.4.2 Transformation of the Advantages of TB PET/CT into Clinical Service Capability

The advantages of fast scanning and low-dose scanning expand the clinical applicability of PET/CT, providing suitable conditions for those who have previously found PET/CT examinations difficult. The fast scan mode enables the maximization of the number of patients examined per unit time, while the combination of fast scans with low or ultra-low doses achieves maximization of the number of patients examined under fixed drug doses. This demonstrates that dynamic scanning provides added value for disease diagnosis.

1.4.3 Preliminary Workflow for TB PET/CT Examinations

In the course of the exploratory clinical application, a preliminary workflow for TB PET/CT examination was established, with a focus on the importance of high-quality and efficient communication and cooperation between each node to maximize operational efficiency. This workflow, which encompasses patient history collection, personalized examination scheme (dynamic or static), injection of imaging agents at individualized doses, individualized acquisition, and image post-processing plan, was designed to prioritize image quality and meet personalized needs, thereby leveraging the advantages of uEXPLORER TB PET/CT to the fullest extent and laying the groundwork for maximizing patient benefits.

1.4.4 Promotion of the Standardized Application of PET/CT Imaging

Through a series of comparative studies with conventional PET/CT, our team has determined the advantages of TB PET/CT and how to circumvent the limitations of conventional PET/CT in clinical practice, thus enabling the full potential of PET/CT to be realized in clinical application. This has provided comprehensive evidence for the revision of clinical application guidelines for PET/CT. Through our team's unremitting efforts, nearly 30 academic papers have been published in this field, including 12 in the *European Journal of Nuclear Medicine and Molecular Imaging* and the *Journal of Nuclear Medicine*, and 13 invited presentations at international academic conferences, which have greatly augmented the recognition of TB PET/CT.

1.4.5 Promotion of Medical-Industry-Research Collaboration

During the exploration of the clinical applications of uEXPLORER TB PET/CT, medical professionals have assessed the performance of the device from the perspective of clinical application and identified issues that need to be addressed, including patent applications. The manufacturing company, with its professional expertise, has addressed the issues raised by medical professionals or incorporated their patents into new device features. The synergistic advantages of the two sides have resulted in mutually beneficial cooperation. The close cooperation between the two sides has expedited the process of product performance validation, optimization, and continuous improvement and has established a novel mode of medical-industrial-research cooperation with multiple implications.

1.5 Outlook for the Clinical Application of TB PET/CT

With the widespread use and continuous exploration of the ultra-long AFOV PET/CT, its numerous potential advantages have been transformed into viable strategies to resolve practical issues in clinical practice. Simultaneously, new challenges have appeared, which necessitated continued exploration. Some of the current salient topics include:

1.5.1 Application in New Drug Development

In recent years, microdosing has emerged as a major focus of drug development. By introducing a minimal amount of novel drugs into the human body to study pharmacokinetics, pharmacodynamics, and drug toxicity, many of the bottlenecks encountered in animal model research have been circumvented. The high sensitivity and whole-body real-time dynamic imaging capabilities of TB PET/CT provide an ideal platform for microdosing research. Real-time dynamic imaging using high-sensitivity TB PET/CT can observe and analyze the distribution of radioactive drugs in various organs and tissues in the body, thereby allowing a comprehensive understanding of the dynamic changes in drug distribution throughout the body. Therefore, the application of TB PET/CT in the field of drug development is highly promising.

1.5.2 Application in Maternal and Fetal Medicine

There remain numerous important issues in the domain of maternal and fetal physiology that require immediate attention, such as the study of oxygen consumption in the maternal and fetal brain, the study of nutrient transfer across the placenta, and the study of fetal infection and inflammation. The remarkable sensitivity of TB PET/CT, in conjunction with ultra-low-dose tracer examination, permits PET imaging to receive radiation doses equivalent to those experienced during intercontinental flights, thereby providing a novel option for research in the specialized field of maternal and fetal medicine.

1.5.3 Multi-Organ Axis Research

There is evidence of a correlation and mutual influence of biological information between multiple organs in the human body. Popular fields of study include the brain–heart axis, the heart–kidney axis, the heart–spleen axis, the liver–spleen axis, and the gut–brain axis. ^{18}F-FDG PET/CT imaging is a common functional imaging examination in clinical practice and is often used to study the mutual influence of multiple organs based on the biological similarity of ^{18}F-FDG to glucose. However, conventional PET/CT is restricted by its limited AFOV and requires multiple bed positions to be collected at different times, thus real-time synchronized biological information between multiple organs cannot be obtained. The extended AFOV of TB PET/CT resolves this issue, allowing the acquisition of real-time matching information among multiple organs. For example, in the multi-organ study of ischemic cardiomyopathy, TB PET/CT can collect biological metabolic information of the heart and other organs simultaneously in a single-bed position, enabling real-time dynamic research on the mutual influence of ischemic effects on the heart and other organs. Therefore, TB PET/CT is promising for the study and application of multi-organ axes.

1.5.4 Low-Dose CT in TB PET/CT

The radiation dose of PET/CT examination is derived from both the radiotracer and CT, where the radiation dose from CT accounts for a larger proportion. The application of ultra-low-dose ^{18}F-FDG PET/CT has been successful in reducing the radiation dose of the radiotracer. However, the main challenge for low-dose PET/CT examination lies in reducing the radiation dose of the CT component.

References

1. Pepin CM. Properties of LYSO and recent LSO scintillators for Phoswich PET detectors. IEEE Trans Nucl Sci. 2004;51:789–95.
2. Surti S, Kuhn A, Werner ME, et al. Performance of Philips Gemini TF PET/CT scanner with special consideration for its time-of-flight imaging capabilities. J Nucl Med. 2007;48(3):471–80.
3. Ng QK, Triumbari EKA, Omidvari N, et al. Total-body PET/CT—first clinical experiences and future perspectives. Semin Nucl Med. 2022;52(3):330–9.
4. Watanabe M, Shimizu K, Omura T, et al. A high-throughput whole-body PET scanner using flat panel PS-PMTs. IEEE Trans Nucl Sci. 2004;51:796–800.
5. Spencer BA, Berg E, Schmall JP, et al. Performance evaluation of the uEXPLORER total-body PET/CT scanner based on NEMA NU 2-2018 with additional tests to characterize PET scanners with a long axial field of view. J Nucl Med. 2021;62(6):861–70.
6. Badawi RD, Shi H, Hu P, et al. First human imaging studies with the EXPLORER total-body PET scanner. J Nucl Med. 2019;60(3):299–303.
7. Prenosil GA, Sari H, Furstner M, et al. Performance characteristics of the Biograph Vision Quadra PET/CT system with a long axial field of view using the NEMA NU 2-2018 standard. J Nucl Med. 2022;63(3):476–84.
8. Nadig V, Herrmann K, Mottaghy FM, et al. Hybrid total-body pet scanners-current status and future perspectives. Eur J Nucl Med Mol Imaging. 2022;49(2):445–59.
9. Xiao J, Yu H, Sui X, et al. Can the BMI-based dose regimen be used to reduce injection activity and to obtain a constant image quality in oncological patients by ^{18}F-FDG total-body PET/CT imaging? Eur J Nucl Med Mol Imaging. 2021;49(1):269–78.
10. He Y, Gu Y, Yu H, et al. Optimizing acquisition times for total-body positron emission tomography/computed tomography with half-dose ^{18}F-fluorodeoxyglucose in oncology patients. EJNMMI Phys. 2022;9(1):45.
11. Yu H, Gu Y, Fan W, et al. Expert consensus on oncological [^{18}F]FDG total-body PET/CT imaging (version 1). Eur Radiol. 2023;33(1):615–26.

2 Comparison of Total-Body PET/CT and Conventional PET/CT

Pengcheng Hu, Zhe Zheng, Runjun Yang, and Xueqi Chen

The limited axial field of view (AFOV) of conventional positron emission tomography/computed tomography (PET/CT), ranging from 15 to 30 cm, restricts the coverage of the body to approximately 1/8 in each bed, thus resulting in a mere 1% of the number of photons emitted by the imaging agent in vivo being effectively detected. This restriction significantly reduces the detection efficiency and sensitivity of the PET system. In contrast, total-body (TB) PET/CT, with an extended AFOV of 194 cm, enables the scanning AFOV to cover the entire body for most patients, significantly increasing the proportion of effective coincidence photons detected. Theoretically, the detection efficiency of TB PET/CT is 40 times that of conventional PET/CT (22 cm AFOV) [1].

TB PET/CT imaging has the theoretical potential to detect smaller lesions or those with lower tracer uptake than conventional PET/CT imaging. However, in clinical practice, various factors can affect image quality, necessitating the optimization of clinical application scenarios and acquisition conditions of TB PET/CT, as well as the exploration and verification of data based on real-world evidence to ensure the maximum benefit for patients. As a novel imaging device, it is also essential to conduct a phantom test to verify its performance before clinical application. Therefore, the center initially explored and verified the performance of the equipment based on phantom data, and then improved, optimized, and verified the preliminary acquisition conditions using clinical data [2].

2.1 Comparison of TB PET/CT and Conventional Digital PET/CT

Before the implementation of new equipment, or after the substitution of certain key components, it is imperative to apply the standard phantom to calibrate and enhance the performance of the equipment. The phantom can be used to examine and verify new equipment, because there are a series of internationally recognized standard parameters for equipment performance, and the performance of the equipment can be objectively evaluated according to the test results [3]. In this study, the constant parameters in the standard phantom were used as the standard to compare and analyze the similarities and discrepancies between TB PET/CT and conventional digital PET/CT for certain key parameters, and the image quality of conventional digital PET/CT under conventional acquisition and reconstruction conditions was employed as the reference. This was done to explore the acquisition conditions of TB PET under the premise of non-inferiority to the conventional digital PET image quality.

P. Hu (✉) · Z. Zheng · R. Yang · X. Chen
Department of Nuclear Medicine, Zhongshan Hospital, Fudan University, Shanghai, China
e-mail: hu.pengcheng@zs-hospital.sh.cn

© Shanghai Scientific and Technical Publishers 2024

H. Shi et al. (eds.), *Total-Body PET/CT*, https://doi.org/10.1007/978-981-97-5065-8_2

The NEMA/IEC NU-2 phantom was employed to compare the background variability (BV), recovery coefficients (RC), and contrast recovery coefficient (CRC) of TB PET/CT (uEXPLORER) and conventional digital PET/CT (uMI 780). The coefficient of variation (COV) of the conventional digital PET/CT in clinical routine settings was utilized as a benchmark to explore the optimal acquisition time and reconstruction parameters of TB PET/CT.

By the standard, the NEMA/IEC NU-2 phantom was injected with 2.65 kBq/mL of radioactive fluid on each occasion, which was equivalent to the average liver activity for a 60-min PET imaging following the injection of ^{18}F-fluorodeoxyglucose (FDG) at 3.7 MBq/kg [4]. Conventional digital PET/CT was reconstructed using the clinical routine settings, while TB PET/CT was reconstructed using varying PET acquisition times and reconstruction parameters [5–8].

From the PET images collected by each PET/CT, three cross-sectional images located in the middle section of the phantom were selected, and three rectangular regions of interest (ROI) with an area of 900 mm^2 were drawn on each cross-sectional image (Fig. 2.1). The COV was then calculated as the standard deviation of each ROI divided by the mean pixel value. The overall COV of the reconstructed image was determined by taking the average value of the COV in the nine ROIs. According to the guidelines of the European Association of Nuclear Medicine Research Ltd. (EARL), an acceptable noise level is indicated by a COV <15%.

For sphere characterization (Fig. 2.2), a cube with a side length of 50 mm was sketched on each sphere in the phantom. The maximum recovery coefficient, RC_{max}, of each spheroid was obtained following the European Association of Nuclear Medicine (EANM) guidelines. The mean recovery coefficient, RC_{mean}, was derived from an additional spherical volume of interest (VOI). In addition, the corresponding CRCs were analyzed according to the NEMA NU-2 2018 standard.

The findings of the phantom study indicated that the cross-calibration of standardized uptake value (SUV) of the background between conventional digital PET/CT and TB PET/CT was

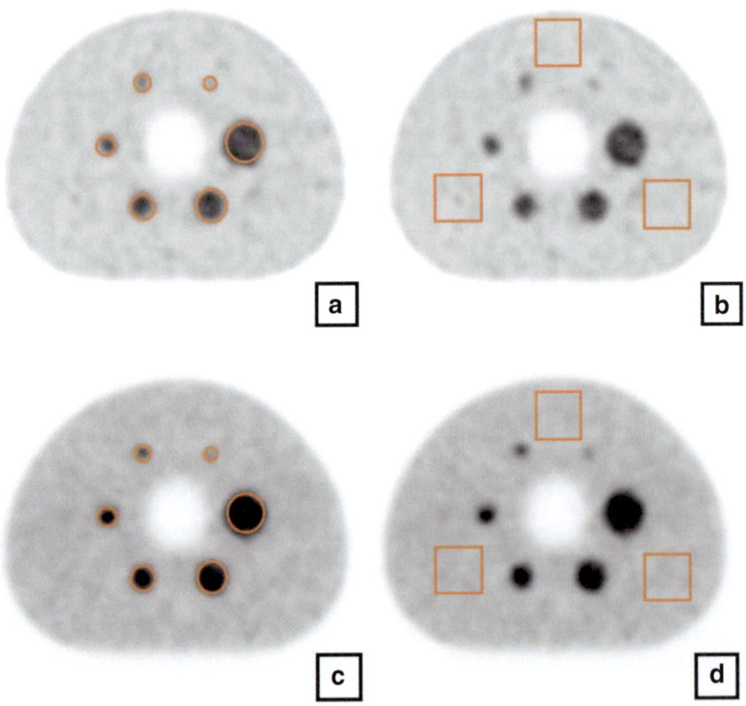

Fig. 2.1 NEMA/IEC NU-2 Phantom Image Analysis. Conventional digital PET (**a**, **b**) and TB PET (**c**, **d**). (**a**) and (**c**) Illustrate the locations of the circular ROIs for the six hot spheres; (**b**) and (**d**) show the locations of the three 900 mm^2 rectangular ROIs used for background COV analysis. The ROIs for conventional digital PET and TB PET were placed in the same locations

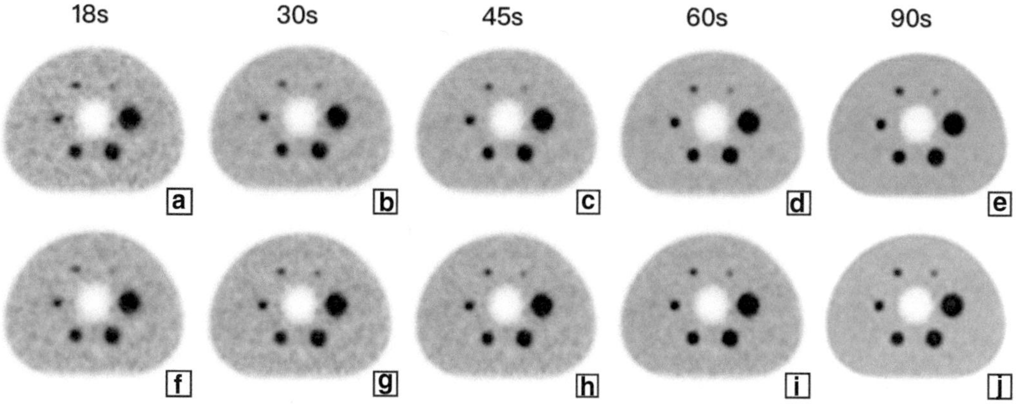

Fig. 2.2 TB PET/CT phantom images for different acquisition durations and different OSEM iterations. (**a**–**e**) Represent two iterations, and (**f**–**j**) represent three iterations. The acquisition times of (**a**) and (**f**) were 18 s. The acquisition times of (**b**) and (**g**) were 30 s. The acquisition times of (**c**) and (**h**) were 45 s. The acquisition times of (**d**) and (**i**) were 60 s. The acquisition times of (**e**) and (**j**) were 90 s. The reconstructed images were derived from all 20 subsets

within the range of 0.95–1.05. It was observed that the noise of the image decreased with the augmentation of the scan duration and the number of iterations. The CRC in the conventional digital PET images was observed to fluctuate slightly because of varying acquisition times, and the CRC in the TB PET was slightly higher than that in the conventional digital PET. The RC_{max} and RC_{mean} of all spheres in both device images were found to be within the EARL limits.

The COV in the conventional digital PET/CT was 11.6% when acquired under the acquisition conditions of clinical routine settings. According to this standard, the acquisition time of TB PET/CT was between 30 and 45 s, and the image quality obtained with two to three iterations was equivalent to that of conventional digital PET/CT in the clinical routine.

To ascertain whether the acquisition time of TB PET/CT for 30–45 s could meet the demands of clinical diagnosis, 40 patients with cancer were subjected to PET/CT imaging. Following the injection of ^{18}F-FDG, PET/CT imaging was performed separately on conventional digital PET/CT and TB PET/CT in random order. To minimize the effect of the delay time between the two PET/CT examinations, those with an interval of more than 40 min were excluded, leaving a total of 30 patients (10 females, 20 males, age 64.2 ± 9.3 years, body mass index 18.1–30.4). The diagnosis included lung cancer (three cases), gastric cancer (five cases), esophageal cancer (three cases), hepatocellular carcinoma (three cases), cholangiocarcinoma (one case), duodenal cancer (one case), pancreatic cancer (two cases), colon cancer (five cases), and rectal cancer (seven cases). No strict exclusion criteria were applied in this study, such as age, diabetes, patient shape, and tumor type, to create a microcosm of real clinical practice with clinical universality.

The reference standard for the conventional digital PET/CT images was acquired at 2–3 min/bed (referred to as G780). To simulate an acquisition time of the 30 s, 45 s, and 60 s, respectively, the PET raw data acquired by TB PET/CT were truncated and reconstructed with two and three iterations, referred to as G30s_2i, G30s_3i, G45s_2i, G45s_3i, G60s_2i, and G60s_3i. A five-point Likert scale was employed to qualitatively assess the image quality, which was also evaluated by liver COV, the target-to-background ratio (TBR), and the signal-to-noise ratio (SNR) [9].

The results demonstrated that TB PET/CT with an acquisition time of 30–45 s and two or three iterations could provide the same image quality as conventional digital PET/CT in routine clinical settings. The inter-reviewer agreement

Kappa value was 0.875, indicating a high degree of consistency between the two reviewers. The qualitative score of G30s_3i in TB PET/CT was lower than the reference value of G780 ($p = 0.001$). However, the other groups with an acquisition time of ≥45 s in TB PET/CT scored higher than G780. In the quantitative analysis, there was no significant difference in the delay time between two scans in different sequences. Additionally, there was no significant difference in liver COV between G780 and G30s_3i PET images ($p = 0.162$) (Fig. 2.3). Thirty-three lesions of the patients were analyzed, and there was no significant difference in TBR between G45s_2i obtained by G780 and TB PET/CT ($p = 0.072$). Moreover, TB PET/CT had a higher lesion SNR than conventional digital PET/CT ($p < 0.001$) (Fig. 2.4).

The phantom and clinical validation studies confirmed that the image quality obtained by TB PET/CT with an acquisition time of 30–45 s and two to three iterations of the ordered subset

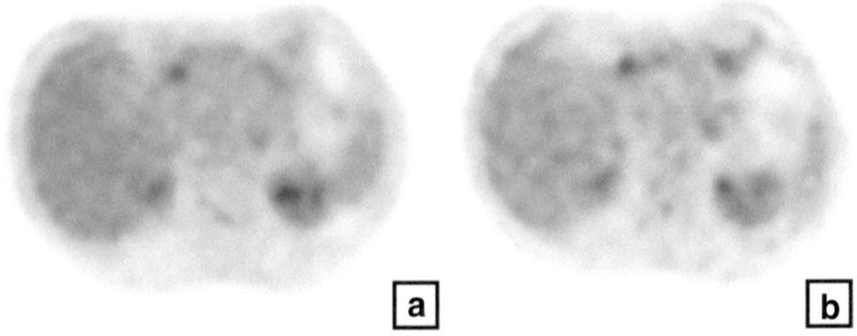

Fig. 2.3 TB PET/CT and conventional digital PET/CT acquisition confirm the diagnostic image quality. Cross-sectional images of a 73-year-old female were obtained by TB PET/CT examination (**a**), followed by a conventional digital PET/CT examination (**b**). The PET images of TB PET/CT were obtained with an acquisition time of 30 s and three reconstruction iterations. The PET acquisition time of 2–3 min in conventional digital PET/CT was reconstructed according to clinical protocols. The noise levels of that two images were comparable and conformed to the requirement of diagnosis

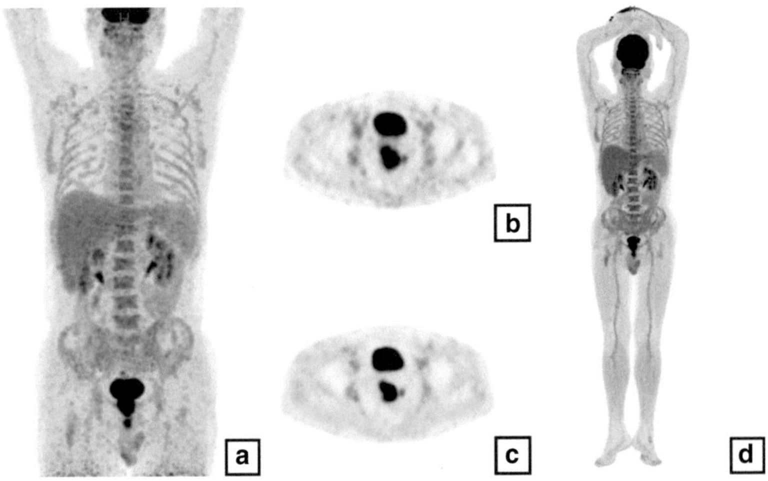

Fig. 2.4 Cross-sectional images of PET and maximum intensity projection (MIP) images of rectal adenocarcinoma. The conventional digital PET images from a 60-year-old male (**a**, **b**) which were reconstructed according to the clinical protocol. TB PET images (**c**, **d**) were acquired for 45 s and reconstructed with two iterations. Axial and coronal TB PET images exhibited satisfactory lesion contrast, meeting the requirements for clinical diagnosis. The sequence of image acquisition was TB PET/CT followed by conventional digital PET/CT

expectation maximization (OSEM) reconstruction algorithm was comparable to that obtained by conventional digital PET/CT under conventional clinical conditions.

2.2 Comparative Analysis of TB PET/CT 2-Min Acquisition Images and Conventional PET/CT Images

The greatly improved sensitivity of TB PET has enabled the implementation of fast scanning. The fast scan is an acquisition mode employed under certain circumstances, where the image quality is not inferior to the conventional PET/CT, but still sufficient to meet the diagnostic requirements, which is not the best performance of TB PET in terms of image quality. In general, high-quality images are still preferred. Therefore, we carried out a comparative analysis of image quality between full-dose ^{18}F-FDG TB PET/CT 2-min acquisition and the conventional digital PET/CT using the conventional acquisition protocols.

A total of 156 patients with pathologically confirmed Hepatocellular carcinoma (HCC) were retrospectively included in this study. The diagnostic performance of the 2-min rapid acquisition of ^{18}F-FDG by TB PET/CT (uEXPLORER) was compared with that of the conventional digital PET/CT (uMI780) with a regular dose. Seventy-eight patients underwent TB PET/CT scans with a total acquisition time of 15 min. The raw data were truncated to 2 min (G2) and 15 min (G15) and reconstructed, respectively, while the other 78 patients underwent the conventional digital PET/CT scan (G780).

The results of the study demonstrated that the primary lesion found in G15 was also found in G2, although three lymph nodes were missed in G2 in comparison to G15. There was no significant difference in the tumor-node-metastasis (TNM) stage of patients among the three groups of G2, G15, and G780. The semi-quantitative parameters such as tumor SUV_{max} and tumor-to-liver ratio (TLR) were comparable among G2, G15, and G780. The receiver operating characteristic (ROC) curve also showed that G2 had good sensitivity to detect liver cancer lesions (Fig. 2.5). In conclusion, TB PET/CT with 2-min acquisition produced comparable diagnostic images to the conventional digital PET/CT for patients with HCC [10].

The preliminary results of this exploratory study were acquired using a small sample and at a single center, which indicated that TB PET/CT (G2 and G15) and conventional digital PET/CT (G780) had similar diagnostic efficacies for liver cancer. To obtain more reliable conclusions, further research with a larger sample size and involving multiple centers is recommended.

A head-to-head comparison of the diagnostic performance of a 106 cm long-axis PET/CT (Biography Vision Quadra PET/CT, Siemens) and the conventional PET/CT (Biography Vision 600, Siemens) was conducted. The results showed that the image quality obtained using the 2-min long-axis PET acquisition was comparable to the standard 16-min conventional PET acquisition. It is noteworthy that while the long-axis PET reconstructed images with the simulated short-time acquisition (0.5 min) were sufficient to detect lesions, the 10-min conventional PET images possessed superior image quality in terms of SNR and TBR.

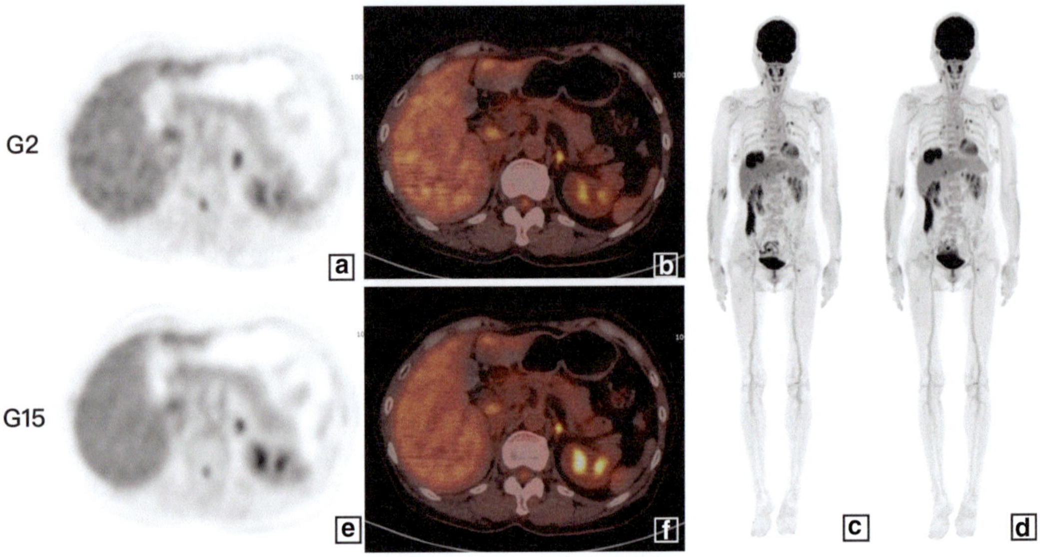

Fig. 2.5 Mixed hepatocellular carcinoma with hilar lymphadenitis. A 77-year-old female was confirmed pathologically to have mixed hepatocellular carcinoma-cholangiocarcinoma and underwent TB PET/CT for staging. The abdominal transverse image, PET/CT fusion image, and PET MIP image are shown in (**a**, **b**, **c**) for G2 and in (**e**, **f**, **d**) for G15, respectively. The lymph nodes were visible in all images, displaying an abnormally high glucose metabolism in the hepatic portal region. Postoperative pathology confirmed the presence of a mixed hepatocellular carcinoma-cholangiocarcinoma, mainly cholangiocarcinoma (90%), with G-III differentiation and hilar lymphadenitis

2.3 Cohort Study of TB PET/CT and Conventional Digital PET/CT in Lesion Detection Efficiency

The use of conventional PET/CT has been found to have limited sensitivity, making it difficult to detect small lesions or those with low uptake of imaging agents. The clinical application of TB PET/CT with long-axis FOV has significantly improved the efficiency of lesion detection. Subjective assessment of the image quality of ^{18}F-FDG TB PET/CT for patients with tumors revealed that the image quality of the 60 s and 30 s acquisitions was acceptable, and that of the 180 s and 120 s acquisitions was excellent. The objective evaluation further demonstrated that the standard deviation of the SUV increased as the acquisition time was shortened; however, the SUV_{max} value of the tumor remained unchanged.

Alberts et al. conducted a comparison of the detection performance of a long-axis PET/CT with 106 cm AFOV (Biography Vision Quadra, Siemens) and a conventional PET/CT with standard AFOV (Biography Vision 600, Siemens). The authors carried out 1-day dual tracer scans with ^{18}F-FDG and either with ^{18}F-prostate-specific membrane antigen (PSMA)-1007 or ^{68}Ga-DOTATOC. The results showed that the long-axis PET/CT 2-min acquisition achieved a comparable SNR, TBR, and image quality to that of the conventional PET/CT 16-min acquisition. Thus, it was concluded that long-axis PET/CT can achieve a similar image quality to that of conventional PET/CT with a shorter acquisition time or a lower dose of radiotracer [11].

TB PET/CT has been explored and verified in clinical practice through the use of half-dose scanning, ultra-low dose scanning, and conventional dose with 30–45 s fast scanning, and the corresponding operational specifications have been established [12]. To further explore the potential advantages of TB PET/CT to identify small lesions or lesions with low tracer uptake, our team designed a head-to-head comparative study of TB PET/CT (uEXPLORER) and the conventional digital PET/CT (uMI 780) to explore the potential lesion detectability of TB PET-CT.

Patients with newly diagnosed tumors were randomly assigned to receive either conventional digital PET/CT (uMI780) or TB PET/CT (uEXPLORER) imaging, following a single injection of the radiotracer. Conventional digital PET/CT was acquired with 2–3 min/bed, denoted as G0. The acquisition time for TB PET/CT was 5 min, and the images were reconstructed sequentially and truncated into 1, 2-, 3-, 4-, and 5-min scans denoted as G1, G2, G3, G4, and G5, respectively. Histopathological findings were used as the diagnostic criteria for primary lesions, lymph node metastases, and partial metastases, while for liver and lung metastases without a pathological diagnosis, magnetic resonance imaging (MRI), and/or contrast-enhanced CT, as well as follow-up imaging, was employed as the diagnostic reference to evaluate the efficiency of PET/CT to detect lesions. Subsequently, two experienced nuclear medicine physicians independently assessed the image quality using a five-point Likert scale and recorded the number of ^{18}F-FDG-positive lesions.

A total of 241 lesions (69 primary lesions; 32 liver, lung, and peritoneal metastases; and 140 regional lymph nodes) in 67 patients with different types of tumors were analyzed. The results showed that the subjective image quality score and SNR increased from G1 to G5, which was significantly higher than that of G0 ($p < 0.05$). Compared with conventional digital PET/CT, G4 and G5 in TB PET/CT detected an additional 15 lesions (two primary lesions; five hepatic, pulmonary, and peritoneal lesions; and eight lymph node metastases) (Figs. 2.6 and 2.7). Compared with conventional

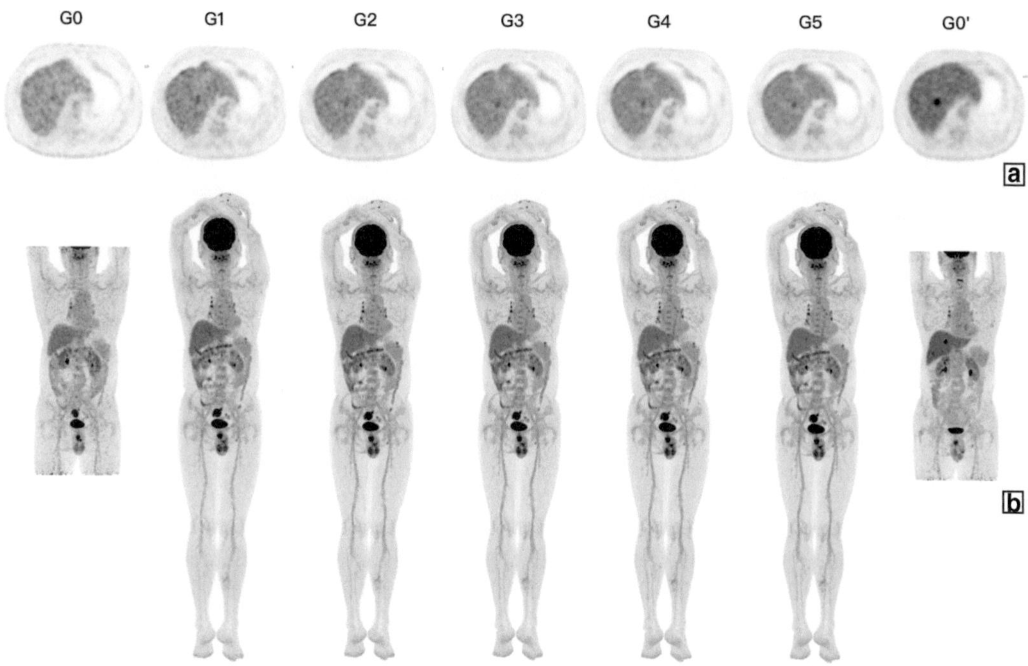

Fig. 2.6 Intrahepatic metastases that were not shown on conventional PET. A 71-year-old male patient with confirmed rectal adenocarcinoma was staged by PET/CT before surgery, with conventional digital PET/CT imaging performed first, followed by TB PET/CT imaging. (**a**) PET cross-sectional images were acquired at different times. (**b**) MIP images of different acquisition duration subgroups. There was no obvious abnormal increase in glucose metabolism in the liver of the G0 group; however, nodular lesions with an abnormal increase in glucose metabolism were present in the liver of the G1–G5 groups. G0′ was the patient's subsequent routine PET/CT (same equipment) imaging after 10 months, which revealed a significant abnormal increase in glucose metabolism, consistent with the location of the lesions shown in the G1–G5 groups

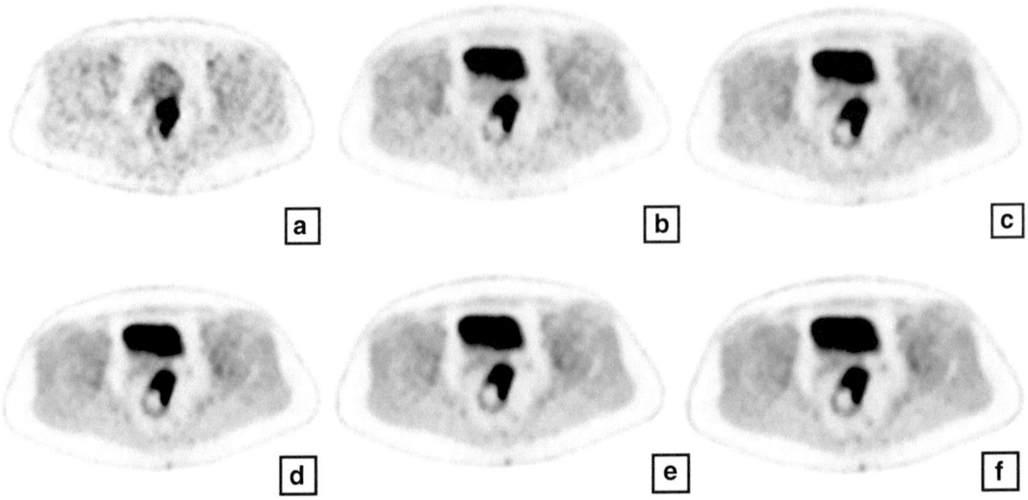

Fig. 2.7 Rectal carcinoma with peripheral lymph node metastasis. A 61-year-old female patient with rectal adenocarcinoma underwent PET/CT for staging. Conventional digital PET/CT was initially performed, followed by TB PET/CT. (**a**) Conventional PET cross-sectional images show an abnormal increase in glucose metabolism in rectal cancer lesions, with no obvious abnormal increase in glucose metabolism in the surrounding area. (**b–f**) Images were reconstructed using TB PET with scanning durations of 1, 2, 3, 4, and 5 min, respectively (the slices were the same as those in (**a**)); only the images with an acquisition time of ≥4 min were able to demonstrate lymph nodes with abnormally high glucose metabolism near the rectum. Postoperative pathology confirmed ulcerative adenocarcinoma of the rectum, invasion of fibrofatty tissue beyond the muscularis propria, and 4/9 lymph node metastasis in the vicinity of the intestines

digital PET/CT, TB PET/CT was found to be more sensitive to detect small lesions (diameter 4.3 mm, SUV_{max} 1.0) or lesions with a low uptake (tumor-to-liver ratio 1.6, SUV_{max} 4.1).

In comparison with conventional PET/CT, TB PET/CT detected 15 additional lesions at G4 and G5 (2 primary lesions; 5 in the liver, lung, and peritoneum; and 8 lymph node metastases). The images reconstructed using the recommended acquisition time (4 min) for TB PET/CT in this study were distinct from the images that used 1 min in our previous study. In the previous study, the 15-min acquisition was used as the standard, rather than pathological diagnosis, which might have resulted in false negatives or false positives. The dose of imaging tracer used in this study (3.7 MBq/kg) was lower than that in the previous study (4.4 MBq/kg). Most importantly, this study employed pathological diagnosis as the gold standard, making the results more objective and reliable.

Image quality and the ratio of target lesions to adjacent normal tissue are important factors that affect the diagnosis of lesions. The present study demonstrated that the lesion SUV_{max} and TLR obtained by G4 in TB PET/CT were significantly higher than those obtained using conventional digital PET/CT (mean SUV_{max} 17.1 and 11.6; mean TLR 7.2 and 5.7, respectively). This increase was attributed to the higher effective count rate and better contrast in normal tissue of TB PET/CT, which improved its ability to detect smaller lesions and those with insignificant uptake of the radiotracer. This study indicated that ^{18}F-FDG TB PET/CT with 4 min of acquisition had a superior lesion detection performance than conventional digital PET/CT, as evidenced by its ability to detect metastatic lymph nodes with a diameter of 4.3 mm and SUV_{max} of 1.0, and low-uptake lesions with a TLR of 1.6 and SUV_{max} of 4.1 in the liver.

References

1. Badawi RD, Shi H, Hu P, et al. First human imaging studies with the EXPLORER total-body PET scanner. J Nucl Med. 2019;60(3):299–303.
2. Hu P, Zhang Y, Yu H, et al. Total-body ^{18}F-FDG PET/CT scan in oncology patients: how fast could it be? Eur J Nucl Med Mol Imaging. 2021;48(8):2384–94.
3. Van Sluis J, De Jong J, Schaar J, et al. Performance characteristics of the digital Biograph Vision PET/CT system. J Nucl Med. 2019;60:1031–6.
4. Chen S, Hu P, Gu Y, et al. Performance characteristics of the digital uMI550 PET/CT system according to the NEMA NU2-2018 standard. EJNMMI Phys. 2020;7(1):43.
5. Gnesin S, Kieffer C, Zeimpekis K, et al. Phantom-based image quality assessment of clinical ^{18}F-FDG protocols in digital PET/CT and comparison to conventional PMT-based PET/CT. EJNMMI Phys. 2020;7(1):1.
6. NEMA standards publication NU 2-2018—performance measurements of positron emission tomography (PET). Rosslyn, VA: National Electrical Manufacturers Association; 2018.
7. Boellaard R, Willemsen AT, Arends B, Visser EP. EARL procedure for assessing PET/CT system specific patient FDG activity preparations for quantitative FDG PET/CT studies. 2013; p. 1–3.
8. Koopman D, van Osch JA, Jager PL, et al. Technical note: how to determine the FDG activity for tumour PET imaging that satisfies European guidelines. EJNMMI Phys. 2016;3(1):22.
9. Zhang Y, Hu P, Wu R, et al. The image quality, lesion detectability, and acquisition time of ^{18}F-FDG total-body PET/CT in oncological patients. Eur J Nucl Med Mol Imaging. 2020;47(11):2507–15.
10. Hu Y, Liu G, Yu H, et al. Diagnostic performance of total-body ^{18}F-FDG PET/CT with fast 2-min acquisition for liver tumours: comparison with conventional PET/CT. Eur J Nucl Med Mol Imaging. 2022;49(10):3538–46.
11. Alberts I, Hünermund JN, Prenosil G, et al. Clinical performance of long axial field of view PET/CT: a head-to-head intra-individual comparison of the Biograph Vision Quadra with the Biograph Vision PET/CT. Eur J Nucl Med Mol Imaging. 2021;48(8):2395–404.
12. Sui X, Liu G, Hu P, et al. Total-body PET/computed tomography highlights in clinical practice: experiences from Zhongshan Hospital, Fudan University. PET Clin. 2021;16:9–14.

3 Clinical Application of Total-Body PET/CT Fast Scan

Yiqiu Zhang, Yibo He, and Hongcheng Shi

Conventional positron emission tomography–computed tomography (PET/CT) scanners typically cover an axial field of view of approximately 15–30 cm and necessitate 5–9 bed positions to acquire a whole-body image (from top of head to mid-thigh). However, with the recommended acquisition speed of 2–3 min/bed position in current guidelines for full-dose (3.7 MBq/kg) ^{18}F-fluorodeoxyglucose (FDG) PET/CT imaging, the total scanning duration can reach 10–30 min. This renders the completion of PET/CT examinations unfeasible for patients who are unable to remain still for prolonged periods of time, and those with limited ability to cooperate.

Theoretically, a 194-cm axial field of view can provide an effective count rate that is 40 times higher than a standard 20-cm axial field of view, which corresponds to a 1/40 reduction in imaging time, while maintaining the signal-to-noise ratio [1]. This would allow for the completion of a total-body PET/CT (TB PET/CT) examination within 15–30 s [2]. As such, we aimed to explore the feasibility of the TB PET/CT (uEXPLORER) fast scanning in real clinical practice.

3.1 Feasibility of ^{18}F-FDG TB PET/CT Fast Scanning

3.1.1 The Fast-Scanning Protocol

The imaging data of 19 patients who underwent ^{18}F-FDG TB PET/CT using the uEXPLORER scanner (United Imaging Healthcare, Shanghai, China) for tumor imaging were analyzed retrospectively [3]. ^{18}F-FDG at 4.4 MBq/kg was administered intravenously 60 min before imaging. Images were acquired in a single bed position with a scanning duration of 15 min. Image reconstruction was first performed on all images, and subsequently on images obtained during the first 180 s (G180), 120 s (G120), 60 s (G60), 30 s (G30), and 18 s (G18) to simulate a fast image acquisition scenario. Image quality was subsequently evaluated by two experienced nuclear medicine physicians using subjective and objective assessment methods.

The results of the study showed that the overall image quality was significantly higher in the G180 and G120 than in the other three groups (all

Y. Zhang · Y. He · H. Shi (✉)
Department of Nuclear Medicine, Zhongshan Hospital, Fudan University, Shanghai, China
e-mail: shi.hongcheng@zs-hospital.sh.cn

© Shanghai Scientific and Technical Publishers 2024
H. Shi et al. (eds.), *Total-Body PET/CT*, https://doi.org/10.1007/978-981-97-5065-8_3

$p < 0.05$), while the difference between the G180 and G120 groups was not significant ($p = 0.21$). We concluded that a 2 min acquisition time provides sufficient information to meet the needs of clinical diagnosis. Taking the image of G900 as a reference, in 109 lesions with a diameter of 6.6–130 mm, the detection rate was 100% in the 180, 120, and 60 s acquisition groups, but was reduced to 91.7% and 78% in the 30 s and 18 s groups, respectively. The reason might be that the acquisition time was too short, resulting in low photon counts and increased noise. In fact, in addition to the acquisition time, the detection rate of lesions also depends on the contrast between the lesion and the surrounding background, the size and shape of the lesion, and the experience of the reader. It is noteworthy that despite the trend for noise increase and imperfect image quality with a short acquisition time, the diagnostic performance remained in the acceptable range for an acquisition time as short as 60 s. We also found that a fast PET protocol with a 30–45 s acquisition time in the TB PET/CT can provide an equivalent image quality as the conventional digital PET/CT (uMI 780, United Imaging Healthcare) with longer clinical acquisition settings [4].

3.1.2 Validation of the Fast-Scanning Program [5]

To verify the feasibility of TB PET/CT fast scanning, a comparative study on the diagnostic outcomes of G30 and G300 images was performed, in which the lowest recommended dose of ^{18}F-FDG (3.7 MBq/kg) was administered [5]. The retrospective study analyzed the data of 88 patients with suspected tumors that were referred to undergo preoperative ^{18}F-FDG TB PET/CT for tumor diagnosis and staging. All patients fasted for at least 6 h before the radiotracer (^{18}F-FDG) was injected at a dose of about 3.7 MBq/kg. The list-mode PET data were acquired over 300 s. The PET images were reconstructed using all 300 s data (G300) and only the initial 30 s (G30). All PET images were reconstructed using an ordered subset expectation maximization algorithm with the following parameters: time of flight (TOF) and point spread function (PSF) modeling; two iterations and 20 subsets; matrix, 192 × 192; slice thickness, 2.89 mm; field of view (FOV), 600 mm (pixel size, 3.125 × 3.125 × 2.89 mm) with a Gaussian post-filter (3 mm). All necessary corrections, such as attenuation and scatter corrections, were applied. A low-dose CT acquisition for attenuation correction was used in the first scan to minimize the radiation exposure of the patients. The low-dose CT acquisition and reconstruction parameters were: 120 kV, 9 mA, spiral pitch factor of 1.0125, 3-mm slice thickness, and 3-mm slice increment. The diagnostic CT acquisition parameters were: 120 kV, tube current modulation, spiral pitch factor of 0.9625, 1-mm slice thickness, 1-mm slice increment. No intravenous or oral contrast agents were used.

The PET/CT image quality was assessed by two nuclear radiologists with 10 years of experience in oncological ^{18}F-FDG PET/CT. The two readers independently assessed the overall G300 and G30 PET image quality using a five-point scale. Images with a score of ≥2 points were considered qualified and acceptable for diagnosis without rescanning. The diagnostic performances of G300 and G30 were measured based on postoperative pathological diagnosis, and the lesions found on PET/CT images but not confirmed by pathology were not included. The two readers assessed the images together and discussed their assessments to reach a consensus. In cases of disagreement, physicians with higher seniority joined the discussion. Each lesion was diagnosed as benign or malignant. The readers were blinded to the patient's history and the reading order was randomized to reduce the memory effect.

According to the postoperative pathological results of the 88 patients, 148 lesions were found in total: 38 benign and 110 malignant. Specifically, 4 benign lesions were found in four patients without malignancies, 1 in each of the patients (1 liver inflammatory pseudotumor, 1 cholecystitis, 1 retroperitoneal paraganglioma, and 1 angiolipoma of the left thigh); and 34 benign lesions (1 liver inflammation, 1 ileocecal inflammatory granuloma, 1 adrenochromocytoma, and 31 pathological lymph inflammation) were from the remaining 84 patients. The 110 malignant lesions found in the 84 patients included 83 primary tumor lesions from 80 patients and 27 metastases from 21 patients, among which 4 metastases originated from previous malignant tumors. Among the 83 primary tumors, 1 patient had stomach and colon primary malignant tumors, 1 had 2 primary lung tumors, 1 had 2 primary colon lesions, and the remaining patients had a single lesion each; 27 in the colorectum, 19 in the lungs, 13 in the stomach, 8 in the liver, 4 in the pancreas, 3 in the esophagus, 2 in the duodenum, and 1 each in the hepatic bile duct, gallbladder, throat, breast, ovary, abdominal cavity (polymorphic undifferentiated sarcoma), and pelvic cavity (papillary urinary epithelial carcinoma). Among the 27 metastases, 3 liver metastases from colon cancer, 2 mesenteric carcinoma nodules from rectal carcinoma, 1 liver metastasis from breast cancer, 1 rectal metastasis from ovarian cancer, 1 brain metastasis from renal cancer, 1 abdominal metastatic carcinoma nodule from pancreatic cancer, and 18 regional lymph node metastases were detected.

The results of the study showed that the average G300 score (4.8 ± 0.4) was significantly higher than that of G30 (2.8 ± 0.7; $p < 0.001$). The weighted kappa values for the inter-observer agreement on the image quality of G300 and G30 were 0.781 (95% confidence interval, 0.614–0.949) and 0.758 (95% confidence interval, 0.637–0.880), respectively. Only two G30 cases were scored as 1 by both readers in this study, and the possible reason for one of the cases was that the patient was overweight, with a body mass of 82 kg, a body mass index (BMI) of 29.4 kg/m^2, and an injected dose of 3.56 MBq/kg. The proportion of G300 and G30 images with acceptable diagnostic quality were similar, at 100% (88/88) and 97.73% (86/88), respectively ($p = 0.497$), which showed that most G30 images could be used for clinical diagnosis. In terms of diagnostic efficiency, the G300 group showed a sensitivity of 89.09%, a specificity of 52.63%, a positive prediction value (PPV) of 84.48%, and a negative prediction value (NPV) of 62.50%, with an overall accuracy of 79.73%. The G30 group showed a corresponding sensitivity of 86.36%, specificity of 52.63%, PPV of 84.07%, and NPV of 57.14%, with an overall accuracy of 77.70%. There was no statistical difference in the diagnostic performance between the two groups.

^{18}F-FDG is not a specific imaging agent for malignant tumors. Some tumors, such as well-differentiated hepatocellular carcinoma, do not accumulate FDG and, therefore, might show false-negative results. For some diseases, such as inflammatory lesions, high FDG uptake could cause false-positive results. Therefore, diagnosis based on ^{18}F-FDG PET/CT imaging relies to some extent on CT imaging and the readers' experience. This study combined the G300 and G30 PET imaging acquisition times with the same spiral CT imaging for PET/CT diagnosis. A higher accuracy rate was obtained using G300 images (79.73%) compared with G30 (77.70%); however, with no statistical significance. Such findings were comparable to those of studies [6–9] on the use of conventional PET/CT, which ranged between 73.8% and 88.9% for the diagnosis of various tumors. Therefore, this supports the clinical feasibility of conventional-dose TB PET/CT with a short acquisition duration of 30 s, provided that image quality is not compromised (Fig. 3.1). Some patients with malignant tumors, especially critically ill patients who do not cooperate well because of pain or other reasons, can benefit from fast PET/CT scanning [10, 11]. However, the longer the acquisition time, the better the image quality when the same dose of ^{18}F-FDG is injected. The high sensitivity of TB PET/CT offers more options for acquisition in clinical practice, and fast scanning is only one of these options, providing more benefit to the appropriate population. Consequently, TB PET/CT fast scanning serves as a promising imaging modality for patients who would otherwise be unable to tolerate prolonged scanning, such as those who are critically ill or in pain.

The European Association of Nuclear Medicine guidelines [12, 13] recommend a linear body mass-based regimen for ^{18}F-FDG PET examinations. The liver signal-to-noise ratio (SNR) of patients with a body mass ≥75 kg would decrease, indicating a degraded image

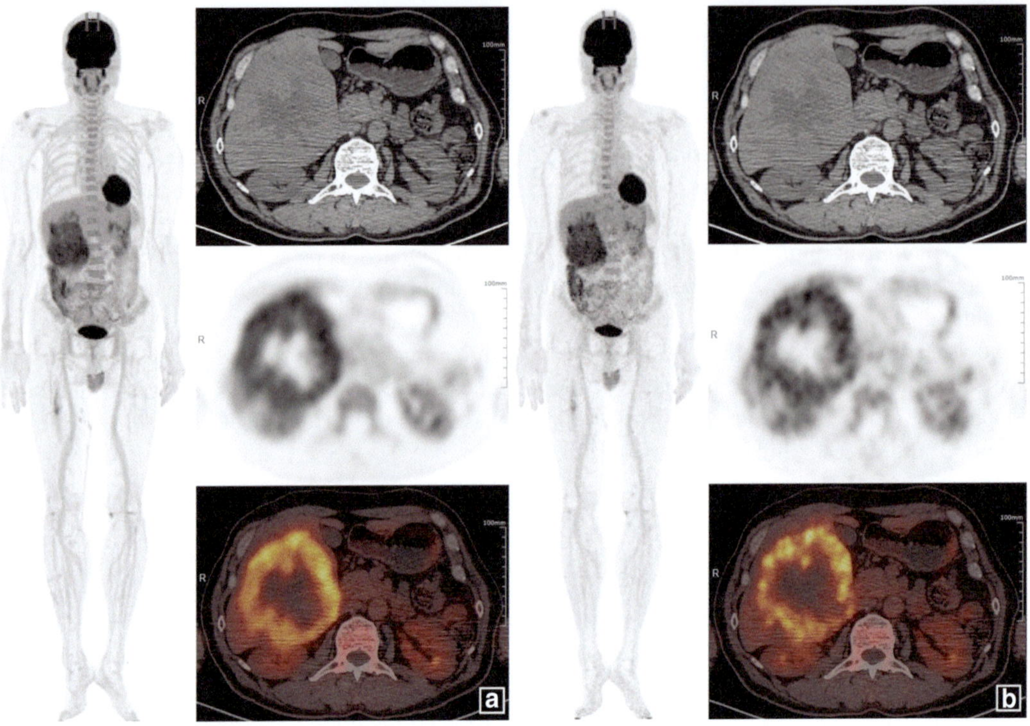

Fig. 3.1 Images of TB PET/CT with acquisition time of 30 s showing liver lesions. A 57-years-old male patient who had a history of hepatitis B found elevated serum alpha-fetoprotein (AFP) that >3000 ng/mL and elevated neuron-specific enolase (NSE) of 19.99 μg/L, when performing physical examination. The other serum tumor markers were normal, including carbohydrate antigen 50 (CA50), CA242, and squamous cell carcinoma antigen. Both abdominal ultrasound and magnetic resonance imaging indicated a diagnosis of primary hepatocellular carcinoma in the right lobe of liver. TB PET/CT images of G300 (**a**) and G30 (**b**) demonstrated the malignant tumor in the right lobe of liver. A grade II hepatocellular carcinoma was eventually confirmed by postoperative pathology

quality because of excessive attenuation and scatter. Our recent research [14] recommended a quadratic relationship between the injected ^{18}F-FDG activity and the patient's BMI and proposed a regimen for total-body PET imaging. The images could be maintained at a constant quality independent of the patient's physique, meeting clinical requirements even with a reduced injected ^{18}F-FDG activity. TB PET/CT 30 s fast acquisition is based on the ^{18}F-FDG full-dose injection scheme recommended by the guidelines of the European Association of Nuclear Medicine; we also detected some residual imaging agent at this patient's injection site, resulting in a lower actual imaging agent dose entering the body than intended, requiring an increase in the acquisition time. Therefore, the acquisition scheme is not immutable, and it needs to be re-optimized in a timely manner according to specific application situations.

3.2 Clinical Application of ^{18}F-FDG TB PET/CT Fast Scanning

3.2.1 Personalization of Image Acquisition Conditions

In the Department of Nuclear Medicine, Zhongshan Hospital, Fudan University, the physician takes a detailed medical history and determines the purpose and focus of the examination before a patient undergoes a PET/CT examination. Based on this, the physician selects the most appropriate PET/CT device from among several available options. The dosage of radiopharmaceuticals and the duration of the scan should be carefully determined according to the status of the patient. For instance, patients requiring imaging of the extremities for conditions such as melanomas, lymphomas, or metastases would largely benefit from an extra-long field of view; children would benefit from a low or ultra-low dose regime; and patients with the inability to remain still would benefit from fast scanning. TB PET/CT also has the advantage that the sequence of PET and CT scans can also be personalized according to the patient's physical condition. The scanning sequence is usually CT localization slice, attenuation correction CT (ACCT), PET acquisition, and diagnostic CT scanning. For instance, in the case of an uncooperative patient, CT might initially be performed for localization and attenuation correction, followed by CT for diagnostic purposes, with PET performed afterwards. This might be followed by an enhanced CT scan if needed. In certain cases, ACCT might be performed in place of diagnostic CT.

3.2.2 Implementation of TB PET/CT Fast Scanning

If the patient cannot be held in a fixed position for a long period of time because of agitation, severe coughing, or pain, the full-dose fast-scanning protocol is preferred. The patient is re-evaluated by the physician in charge of medical safety and scanning protocol confirmation before the examination. The aim is to ensure patient safety during the examination and to obtain good image quality that meets diagnostic needs. Under routine circumstances, patients are recommended to be positioned with both hands behind the head. However, in the case of suspected lesions on the upper extremities, both arms should be placed along the sides of the body, or across the chest. In terms of the scanning sequence, a CT localization scan can be performed first, followed by ACCT and PET to determine the extent of coverage for diagnostic CT imaging. A standard coverage from the top of the skull to mid-thigh would be sufficient in the absence of suspected lesions in the lower extremities. The duration of the PET scan is routinely preset to 3 min, and can be prematurely terminated depending on the patient's condition. In terms of patient positioning, the "go with the flow" approach can be adopted to prioritize patient comfort (Fig. 3.2). If the patient cannot tolerate the completion of the examination during the acquisition process, the PET examination can be interrupted at any time, and if the patient does not shift during the acquisition process, PET image reconstruction can be performed according to the completed duration (Fig. 3.3). In the case of critically ill patients, or those who are unsuitable for diagnostic CT following failure of a PET scan, diagnosis can be made based on a fusion of ACCT and PET images (Fig. 3.4).

In critically ill patients from the emergency department with no suspicious bilateral lower extremity lesions in the history, a diagnostic CT might be performed before PET. The diagnostic CT scan is routinely performed from the top of the skull to the mid-thigh, and then a fast PET scan is routinely preset for 2 min or even less (Fig. 3.5). The advantage is that when a patient encounters an unexpected situation during a PET scan and needs to terminate the examination, the PET data already acquired can be used for reconstruction and can also be fused with diagnostic CT for clinical diagnosis.

3.2.3 Selection of High-Quality Images of Reconstruction from TB PET/CT Long Duration Acquisition Images

Longer scanning durations are known to yield better image quality, provided that radiopharmaceutical tracer administration is constant. In clinical practice, for patients injected with regular doses of ^{18}F-FDG, if the patient is in good general condition and can fully cooperate with the examination, a 5 min acquisition is routinely chosen to achieve the best image quality (Fig. 3.6). If the patient moves significantly during the image acquisition, a short-time acquisition image can be preferen-

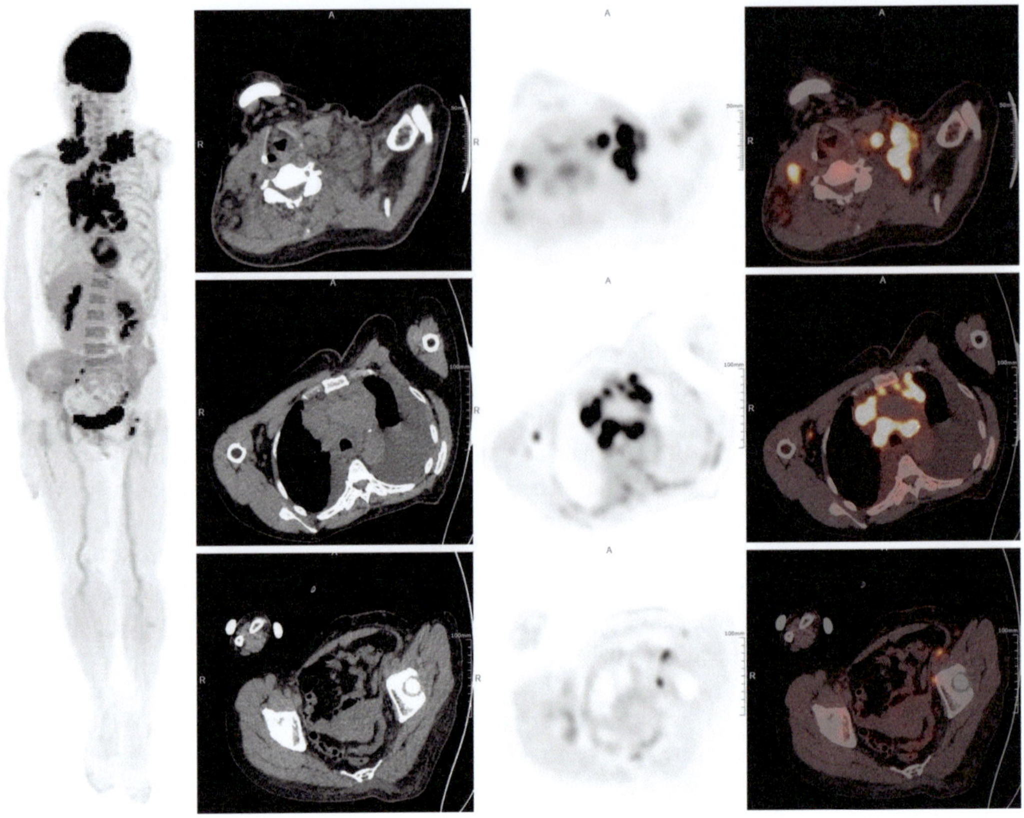

Fig. 3.2 Fast-scanning TB PET/CT images of patient in a compulsive position. A 64-years-old female patient had been diagnosed peripheral T-cell lymphoma (the non-specific type). She was unable to lie supine for a prolonged period of time; therefore, full-dose fast-scanning PET/CT imaging protocol with preset time of 3 min for PET scanning was applied to this patient in a compulsive lateral position, with a scanning order of CT scout, ACCT, PET, and diagnostic CT. TB PET/CT images demonstrated lymphomas involving lymph nodes in areas of the bilateral neck, the clavicular region, the axillary fossa, the mediastinum, the bilateral lung hila, the pelvis, and the left inguina

tially selected to meet the diagnostic needs by selecting different time windows for image reconstruction; if the examination is terminated because of a special condition of the patient during image acquisition, the reconstructed image can be preferentially selected from the acquired information to meet the diagnostic requirements (Fig. 3.7).

In summary, the fast acquisition or short reconstruction of full-dose ^{18}F-FDG TB PET/CT images in no less than 30 s expands the ability of nuclear medicine to serve the clinical setting, enabling the examination of patients who are critically ill or unable to lie for a long time based on a personalized TB PET/CT scanning. For patients who move during the examination, the images can be reconstructed in a short period of time to meet the diagnostic needs, ensuring a benefit to the patient.

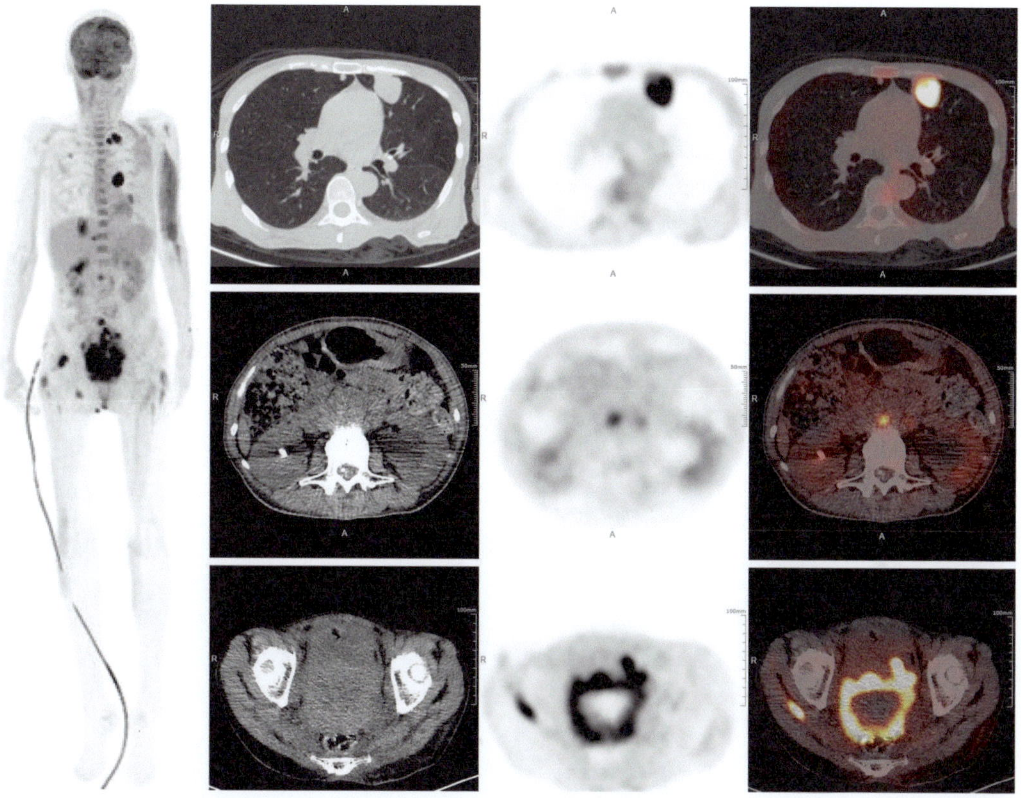

Fig. 3.3 TB PET/CT images acquired only for 87 s. A female 47-years-old patient, who had a history comprehensive chemoradiotherapy for cervical cancer, presented with auditory and visual hallucinations secondary to cerebral hemorrhage caused by an accidental fall 2 weeks ago. She was given symptomatic treatment in the emergency room since the accident. Since tolerance to standard PET/CT scanning could not be guaranteed for this patient, a fast-imaging protocol of 3 min was preset for PET scanning. Eventually, the patient was only scanned for 87 s when she complied that she could not tolerated anymore. The TB PET/CT images indicated a diagnosis of cervical cancer invading the uterine body, the bladder, and the lower segments of bilateral ureters with associated hydronephrosis, in companied with abdominopelvic implantation metastases, retroperitoneal lymph node metastases, and bilateral lung metastases

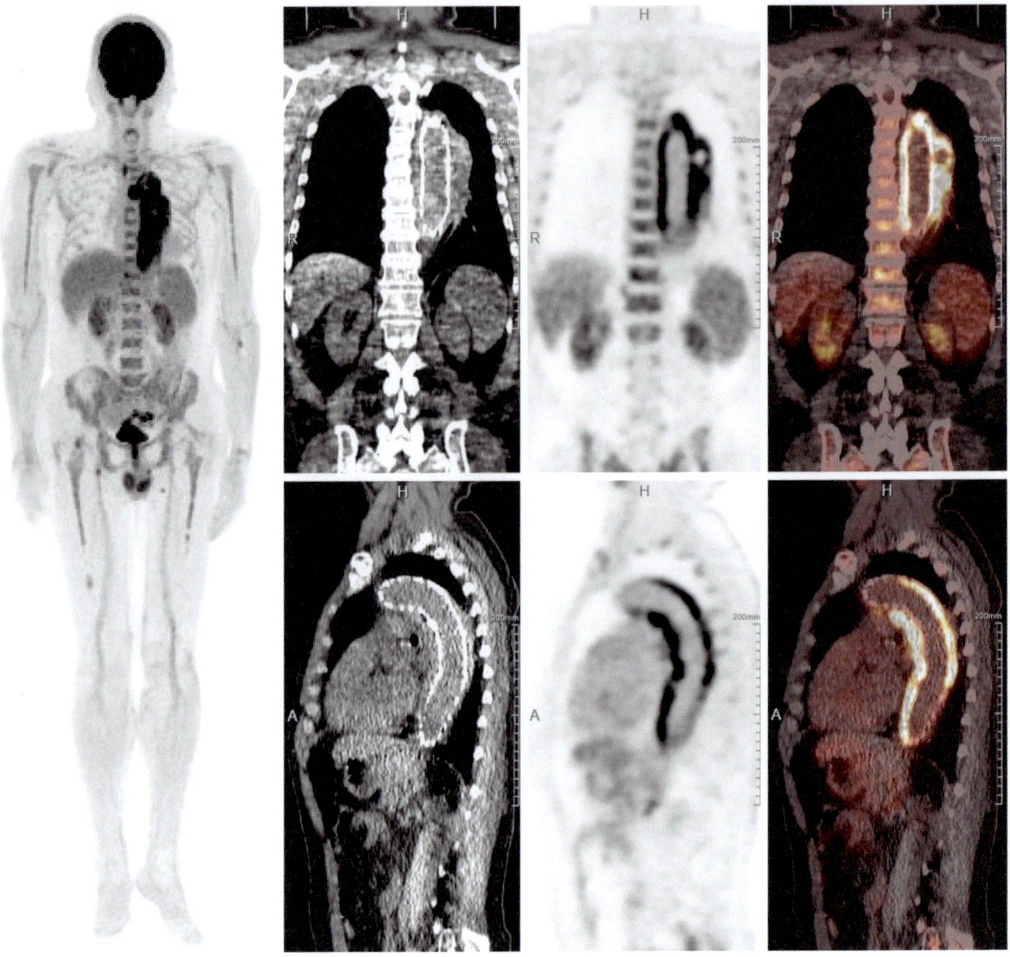

Fig. 3.4 Fast-scanning TB PET/CT images of a critically ill patient. A male patient of 57 years old admitted with intermittent hemoptysis, after two times of stent implantation for dissection of aorta. PET/CT scanning was performed to this patient in a scheduled scanning order of CT scout, ACCT, PET, and diagnostic CT. Despite a preset 3 min for PET scanning, only a duration of 93 s could be tolerated by this patient, and thus the diagnostic CT scan was not feasible. The diagnosis was made with PET/ACCT fused images, which indicated a potential aortic dissection-esophageal fistula with inflammation of the aortic wall adjacent to the stent

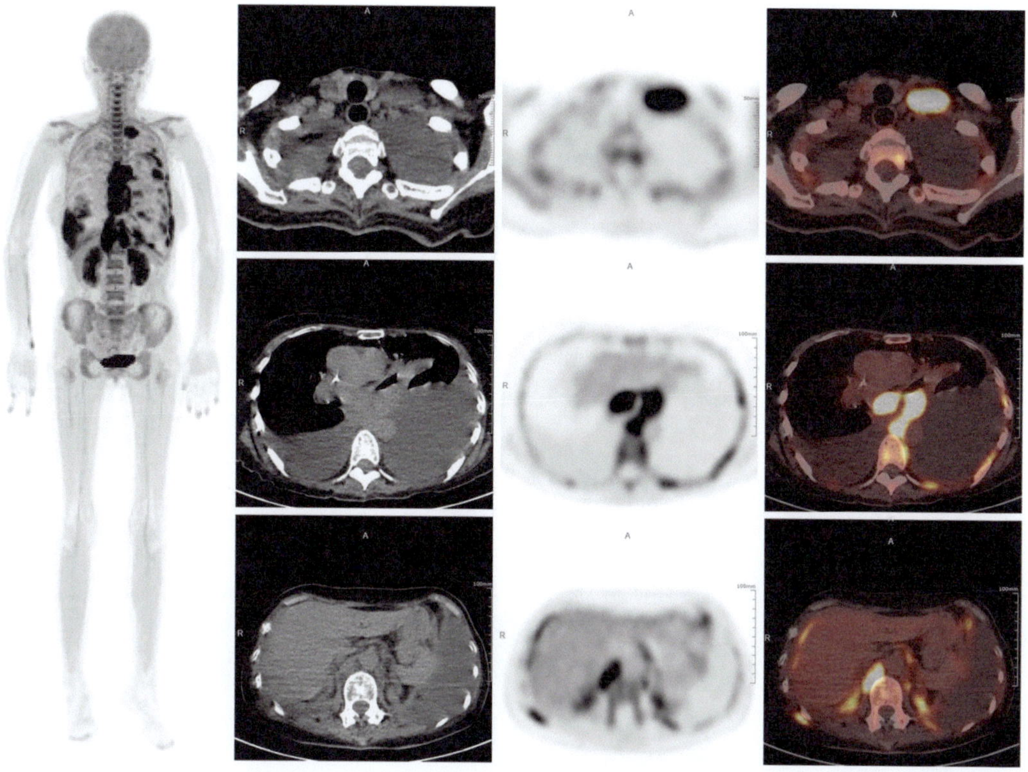

Fig. 3.5 Fast 2-min TB PET/CT images in an emergency setting. A female patient of 59 years old was confirmed lymphoma by biopsy pathologies of left cervical lymph node and bone marrow 3 months ago. Baseline PET/CT revealed lymphomas involving lymph nodes in the middle to posterior mediastinum, the bilateral lung hila, the left neck root, the bilateral clavicular regions, bilateral post-diaphragmatic-crura spaces, the retroperitoneum, the pelvis, and the bilateral inguinal, as well as left mid-superior humeral intramedullary cavity and the right margin of the second lumbar vertebrae. An efficacy evaluation was proposed after three courses of chemotherapy. The patient presented to the emergency room after half a month of poor appetite and post-prandial vomiting, and was evaluated using TB PET/CT. A fast-scanning protocol of PET/CT with preset 2 min for PET scanning was arranged to this patient. The examination was completed in the scanning order of CT scout, ACCT, diagnostic CT, and PET. The TB PET/CT images demonstrated a reduction in size of the lesions in the middle to posterior mediastinum, with reduced glucose metabolism, but was still metabolic active; bilateral pleural involvement was newly discovered; progression was found in lesions of lymph nodes in the left clavicular region, bilateral post-diaphragmatic-crura spaces, and the hepatogastric space; while regressions of pathological lymph nodes were visualized in other regions, including the neck and clavicular region, the space between the superior vena cava and the trachea, the retroperitoneum, the mesenteric root, the pelvis, and the bilateral inguinal regions; lesions in the left upper humeral medullary cavity and the right margin of the second lumbar vertebrae disappeared

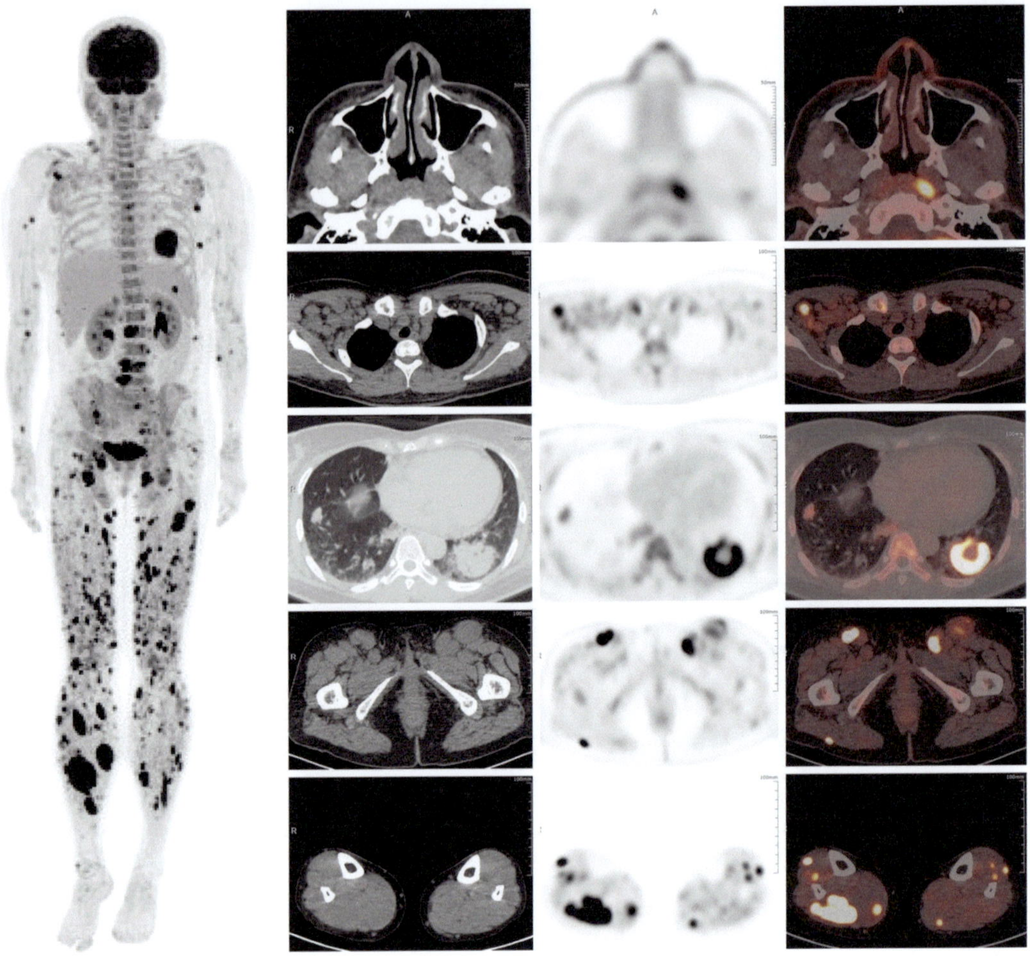

Fig. 3.6 TB PET images with acquisition duration of 5 min. A female patient of 55 years old admitted with a 5-year history of subcutaneous nodules, which were recently found to progress in size and number. Since lesions were suspected in the four limbs, TB PET/CT was performed to this patient. The general condition of this patient was good, thus an acquisition time of 5 min was preset for PET scanning. The PET/CT scanning was completed in the scanning order of CT scout, ACCT, diagnostic CT, and PET. The TB PET/CT images showed lymphomas involving multiple lymph nodes over the entire body, the nasopharynx, the tongue, the left breast, bilateral lungs, the abdominopelvic peritoneum, the subcutaneous soft tissues and muscles, and multiple bones with pathological fractures in the second and fourth lumbar vertebrae

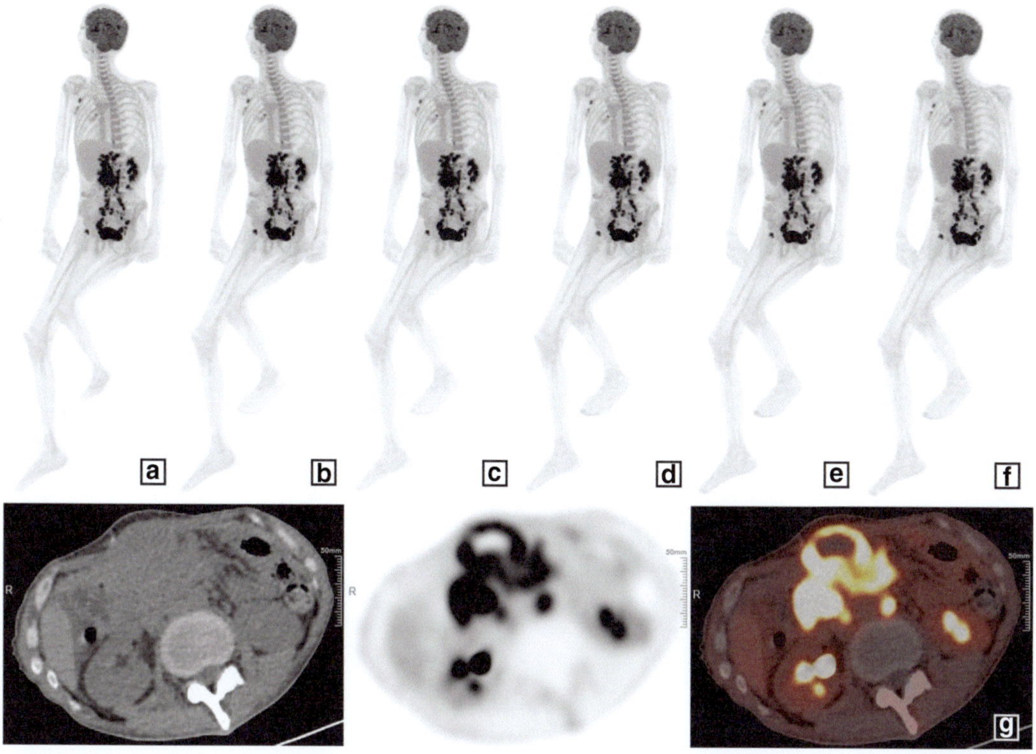

Fig. 3.7 Reconstructed short-time TB PET images from a patient with movement. A male patient, of 39 years old, received chemotherapy combined with targeted drug therapy, after abdominal tumor resection and partial gastrointestinal resection, because of low differentiated abdominal adenocarcinoma. She was scheduled for re-staging with PET/CT. An acquisition time of 3 min was preset for the PET scanning, but the patient moved significantly during the examination (**a**). TB PET/CT was scanned in the order of CT scout, ACCT, diagnostic CT, and PET. No significant movement artifact was visualized in images reconstructed from the first 90 s (**b**), 75 s (**c**), 60 s (**d**), 45 s (**e**), and 30 s (**f**) of acquisition time. As such, PET images with acquisition time of 90 s (**b** and **g**) were used for diagnosis. The TB PET/CT images indicated local recurrence in the abdominal cavity with distant metastases to the abdominopelvic cavity, the lymph nodes of in the abdominopelvic cavity, the retroperitoneal space, the post-diaphragm-crura space, the right internal mammary region, and the right axillary, as well as metastases to the left lung

References

1. Badawi RD, Shi H, Hu P, et al. First human imaging studies with the EXPLORER total-body PET scanner. J Nucl Med. 2019;60(3):299–303.
2. Cherry SR, Jones T, Karp JS, et al. Total-body PET: maximizing sensitivity to create new opportunities for clinical research and patient care. J Nucl Med. 2018;59(1):3–12.
3. Zhang Y, Hu P, Wu R, et al. The image quality, lesion detectability, and acquisition time of ^{18}F-FDG total-body PET/CT in oncological patients. Eur J Nucl Med Mol Imaging. 2020;47(11):2507–15.
4. Hu P, Zhang Y, Yu H, et al. Total-body ^{18}F-FDG PET/CT scan in oncology patients: how fast could it be? Eur J Nucl Med Mol Imaging. 2021;48(8):2384–94.
5. Zhang Y, Hu P, He Y, et al. Ultrafast 30-s total-body PET/CT scan: a preliminary study. Eur J Nucl Med Mol Imaging. 2022;49(8):2504–13.
6. Crivellaro C, De Ponti E, Elisei F, et al. Added diagnostic value of respiratory-gated 4D ^{18}F-FDG PET/CT in the detection of liver lesions: a multicenter study. Eur J Nucl Med Mol Imaging. 2018;45(1):102–9.
7. Kim JY, Kim MH, Lee TY, et al. Clinical role of ^{18}F-FDG PET-CT in suspected and potentially operable cholangiocarcinoma: a prospective study compared with conventional imaging. Am J Gastroenterol. 2008;103(5):1145–51.
8. Taralli S, Scolozzi V, Foti M, et al. ^{18}F-FDG PET/CT diagnostic performance in solitary and multiple pulmonary nodules detected in patients with previous cancer history: reports of 182 nodules. Eur J Nucl Med Mol Imaging. 2019;46(2):429–36.

9. Kubiessa K, Purz S, Gawlitza M, et al. Initial clinical results of simultaneous 18F-FDG PET/MRI in comparison to ^{18}F-FDG PET/CT in patients with head and neck cancer. Eur J Nucl Med Mol Imaging. 2014;41(4):639–48.
10. Nardo L, Schmall JP, Werner TJ, et al. Potential roles of total-body PET/computed tomography in pediatric imaging. PET Clin. 2020;15:271–9.
11. Zhao YM, Li YH, Chen T, et al. Image quality and lesion detectability in low-dose pediatric ^{18}F-FDG scans using total-body PET/CT. Eur J Nucl Med Mol Imaging. 2021;48(11):3378–85.
12. Delbeke D, Coleman RE, Guiberteau MJ, et al. Procedure guideline for tumor imaging with ^{18}F-FDG PET/CT 1.0. J Nucl Med. 2006;47(5):885–95.
13. Boellaard R, Delgado-Bolton R, Oyen WJ, et al. FDG PET/CT: EANM procedure guidelines for tumour imaging: version 2.0. Eur J Nucl Med Mol Imaging. 2015;42(2):328–54.
14. Xiao J, Yu H, Sui X, et al. Can the BMI-based dose regimen be used to reduce injection activity and to obtain a constant image quality in oncological patients by ^{18}F-FDG total-body PET/CT imaging. Eur J Nucl Med Mol Imaging. 2021;49(1):269–78.

4 Application of Total-Body PET/CT in Evaluation of Radiotracer Biodistribution in Human

Guobing Liu and Hongcheng Shi

One of the advantages of positron emission tomography–computed tomography (PET/CT) lies in its ability to quantify the in vivo distribution, metabolism, and clearance of the tracer, from which a series of pathophysiological processes of tumor metabolism can be revealed at the molecular level, for example, tumor metabolism, blood perfusion, proliferation, receptor expression, and the binding between the ligand and receptor. 2-[^{18}F]Fluoro-2-deoxy-D-glucose (^{18}F-FDG) PET/CT imaging and its semiquantitative parameter, standardized uptake value (SUV), have played a significant role in the diagnosis and treatment of tumors and thus have been widely used. However, the static imaging acquired over a relatively long time (about 60 min) after tracer administration can only provide limited information from single time point of whole tracer metabolism. In contrast, dynamic PET imaging allows for the quantitative assessment of the characteristics of the key steps regarding blood perfusion, delivery, tissue uptake, retention, and release of the tracer, and thus can non-invasively represent the whole process of tumor metabolism, which would facilitate to the accurate treatment and diagnosis of the tumor.

Based on dynamic PET/CT imaging, the evaluation of pharmacokinetic parameters of radiopharmaceuticals has many values. First, it shows how tracers get to the target point and reveals the biological characteristics of diseases. Taking ^{18}F-FDG PET as an example, the kinetic parameters allow the measurement of both the rate of tracer delivery to cancer cells and the rate of its metabolism, demonstrating a balance or imbalance between substrate delivery and utility. This information might predict important outcomes, such as the therapeutic response and survival of patients with tumors [1]. Second, tracer kinetic analysis provides more precise interpretations of PET images. For example, the retention of ^{18}F-FDG in tumor tissues at notable concentrations remains for several hours after injection. As such, static tumor images at the typical 1-h-postinjection time point reflect a mixture of unmetabolized ^{18}F-FDG and ^{18}F-FDG-6-P trapped by tumors, and static PET imaging cannot distinguish these two compounds. Dynamic imaging and kinetic analysis, however, can use the time course of radioactive ^{18}F-FDG in the blood and the total ^{18}F-FDG plus ^{18}F-FDG-6-P in the tissue to infer the rate of intracellular ^{18}F-FDG-6-P accumulation and provide a more specific estimate of tumor glucose metabolism. It has been reported that this technique could be applied to measure therapeutic response [1, 2]. Third, kinetic analysis can help avoid pitfalls in interpreting standard clinical static uptake images. For example, for some tumors with high glucose metabolic rates, the trapping of tracer as ^{18}F-FDG-6-P might persist over time. Thus, a marked change in the SUV can

G. Liu · H. Shi (✉)
Department of Nuclear Medicine, Zhongshan Hospital, Fudan University, Shanghai, China
e-mail: shi.hongcheng@zs-hospital.sh.cn

© Shanghai Scientific and Technical Publishers 2024
H. Shi et al. (eds.), *Total-Body PET/CT*, https://doi.org/10.1007/978-981-97-5065-8_4

be caused by a small change in scanning time around 1 h after injection. Therefore, variability of uptake time in serial scans can considerably confound the assessment of therapeutic response. In contrast, kinetic analysis avoids this pitfall. Finally, kinetic analysis is helpful to determine the optimal imaging time of a specific tracer for a specific tumor.

The axial field of view (AFOV) of traditional PET/CT is about 15–30 cm. Therefore, simultaneous total-body dynamic imaging is unavailable for this kind of equipment, and thus cannot meet the basic requirement of pharmacokinetics. In recent years, the advent of PET/CT scanners with long AFOVs, represented by the "uEXPLORER" (AFOV: 194 cm; United Imaging Healthcare, Shanghai, China) [3] and the "Quadra" (AFOV: 106 cm, Siemens Healthineers, Knoxville, TN, USA) [4], has laid the foundation for pharmacokinetic analysis.

4.1 Introduction to the Theory of Pharmacokinetics in Traditional Clinical Pharmacology

The main task of traditional clinical pharmacology is to investigate the interaction rules between a drug and the human body, including pharmacodynamics (PD) and pharmacokinetics (PK). PD mainly deals with the effect of the drug on the body and the underlying rules, to determine the mechanism of drug for prevention and treatment of diseases. PK determines how the body disposes of the drug and its dynamic change over time, including drug absorption, distribution, biotransformation (or metabolism) and clearance, especially the dynamic change in its concentration in blood over time. In this section, we briefly introduce the key concepts of PK in relation to the kinetic analysis of PET images.

4.1.1 Key Theoretical Points Regarding the Compartment Model in Clinical Pharmacology

4.1.1.1 Compartment Model

The core principle of clinical pharmacology is that the drug will not exert its pharmacological action and exhibit the corresponding effect on the body until it reaches a certain concentration, which keeps changing with the absorption, distribution, metabolism, and clearance over time. The kinetic analysis of a drug can be carried out using the compartment model method and non-compartment model method. As the latter is always associated with a complicated algorithm, it will not be introduced here. In the compartment model, the organic body is considered as a system, where multiple compartments are divided according to the dynamic characteristics of the drug. The compartment is a hypothetical space, which is not associated with any exact anatomy and physiological function. The areas of the body that possess an equal or similar delivery rate of drug are taken as one compartment. In most cases, the drug can get in and out of the compartment; therefore, it is commonly called an open compartment system.

The open compartment system often includes two types, namely:

1. **Open one compartment model**: If the drug reaches a balance among different parts of the body instantaneously after administration, i.e., the concentration of drug between the blood and tissue can achieve equilibrium quickly, the system can be regarded as a one compartment model, as shown in Fig. 4.1a. In this figure, D denotes drug absorption, K_a is the constant of the absorption rate, C represents the blood concentration of the drug, V_d is the apparent distribution volume, CV_d is the total amount of drug in the body, K_e is the con-

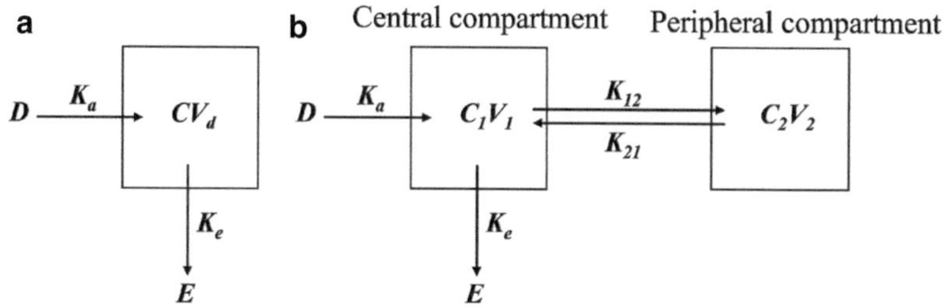

Fig. 4.1 Diagrammatic sketch of open compartment model system. (**a**) The open one compartment model. (**b**) The open two compartment model

stant of clearance rate, while E denotes the cleared amount of the drug.

2. **Open two compartment model**: Most of the time, the concentration of the drug between the blood and tissue can achieve equilibrium quickly in one part of the body, but not in another part, where the delivery rates of drug are close to each other. The former area can be taken as central compartment, which always comprises organs or tissues with a full blood supply, such as the kidney, brain, heart, and liver. The latter area in which equilibrium is always delayed is regarded as a peripheral compartment, like the muscle, the skin, and the fat, which lacks a blood supply, or commonly has slow blood flow. This kind of compartment system is called a two compartment model, as show in Fig. 4.1b. In this figure, transfer of the drug between the central and peripheral compartments is reversible, with K_{12} and K_{21} indicating the first-order constant rate of drug transfer forward and back from the central compartment to the peripheral compartment, respectively. When equilibrium is achieved between these two compartments, their constant rates are equal to each other, namely, $K_{12} = K_{21}$. Most drugs are delivered and distributed in accordance with the two compartment mode.
3. **Open three compartment model and other complicated compartment models**. If the delivery rate of a drug within the peripheral compartment still differs dramatically, a three compartment model is considered, as shown in Fig. 4.2a. Besides, pharmacokinetics of some drugs even comply with more complicated compartment models. For example, although the delivery characteristics of some drugs comply with the two compartment model, they are cleared not only through the central compartment, but also through the peripheral compartment, as shown in Fig. 4.2b. However, some drugs that are characterized by the two compartments or three compartment models can be cleared only through the peripheral compartment (Fig. 4.2c, d). The abovementioned compartment models only apply to drugs that are administered intravenously. For drugs that are not administered intravenously, for example, oral administration, it should be absorbed through a peripheral compartment before arriving in the central compartment, and then distributed and metabolized through a one compartment model or two compartment model, while the unabsorbed drug is cleared through a peripheral compartment (Fig. 4.2e).

It should be noted that the "compartment" is neither an exact anatomy space nor a specific kinetic parameter. Many factors, such as the sampling pattern and the method used for testing the drug concentration, would affect the determination of the compartment model. Therefore, the non-compartment model has actually been commonly used in clinical practice.

4.1.1.2 Distribution and Clearance

For most of drugs, blood concentration-time curves always decays in a biexponential way, including two phases and complying with characteristics of a two compartment model distribution.

1. **Distribution phase**: Also called the α phase, this corresponds to the rapid decrease period of the blood drug concentration. This phase always indicates fast delivery of the drug through the

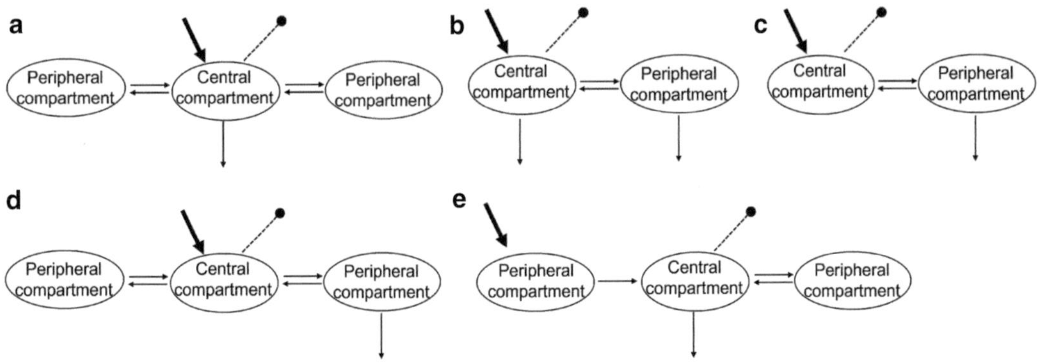

Fig. 4.2 Diagrammatic sketch of multiple compartment model systems. Thick black arrows indicate drug administration, while the dashed line with a round dot indicates sampling. (**a**) Typical three compartment model. (**b**) Two compartment model with drug cleared both from central compartment and peripheral compartment. (**c**) Two compartment model with drug cleared only from peripheral compartment. (**d**) Three compartment model with drug cleared only from one peripheral compartment. (**e**) Three compartment model with drug absorbed through a peripheral compartment and cleared from the central compartment

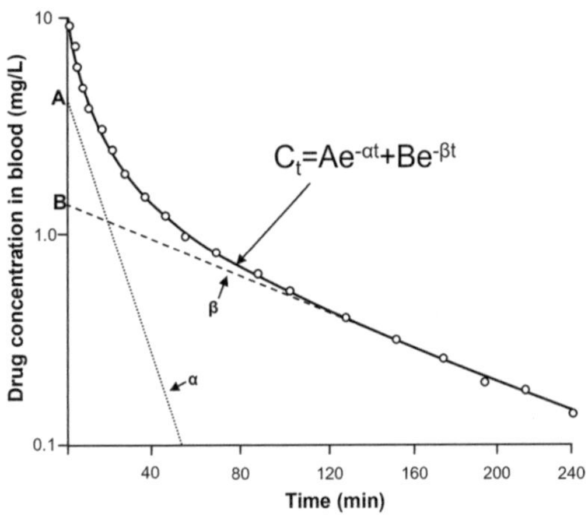

Fig. 4.3 Drug concentration-time curve of veinous-drug and calculation of the corresponding parameters. α is the constant of the distribution rate, and β is the constant of the clearance rate

blood flow into the central compartment, followed by distribution to the peripheral compartment, with only a little cleared by metabolism and excretion. This phase is mainly associated with drug distribution, and is thus called the distribution phase, with α denoting the constant rate of distribution (Fig. 4.3).

2. **Clearance phase**: Also called the β phase, this corresponds to the period in which the drug distribution gradually achieves equilibrium. The decrease in the blood drug concentration in this phase always indicates clearance of the drug from the central compartment. Under the rules of maintaining dynamic equilibrium, the concentration of the drug in the peripheral compartment decreases in portion to the concentration of the drug in the blood. Therefore, the shape of this phase is similar to a straight line, in which β denotes the constant rate of clearance.

   The whole kinetic process of a two compartment model can be reflected by the following formula:

$$C_t = A\mathrm{e}^{-\alpha t} + B\mathrm{e}^{-\beta t}$$

   where C_t is the blood concentration of the drug at time t, α is the constant of the distribution rate, and β is the constant of the clearance rate. B is the intercept when the segment of the β phase of the drug concentration-time curve is extended to the longitudinal ordinate (drug concentration). When subtracting the tested plasma drug concentration from the corresponding value on the curve in the segment of the β phase, and then drawing a line that connects all the calculated differences in the same coordinates, extension of the line to the longitudinal ordinate will get an intercept, namely A (Fig. 4.3). A and α, as well as B and β, can be calculated through least squares regression.

4.1.1.3 Clearance Kinetics

1. **First-order clearance kinetics**: This means that the proportion of the cleared drug is consistent over time, namely, the amount of cleared drug within a unit time is proportional

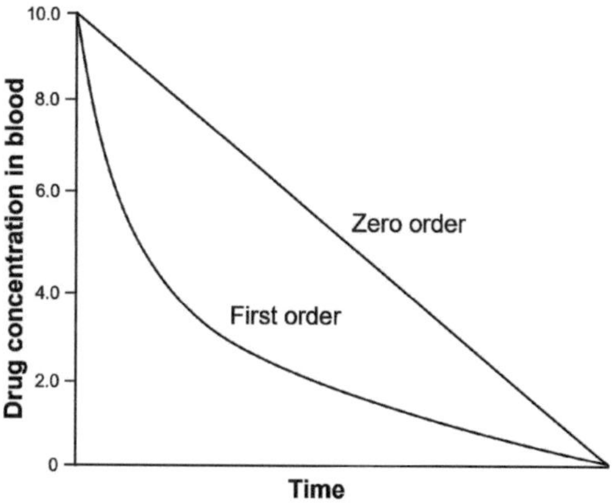

Fig. 4.4 Diagrammatic sketch of a drug concentration-time curve that complies with first-order or zero-order clearance kinetics

to the concentration of the drug in blood. The drug concentration-time curve that complies with first-order clearance kinetic is presented as a curve (Fig. 4.4).

For most drugs, their clearance complies with first-order clearance kinetics, and their half-life time is a constant. First-order clearance kinetic can be described using the following formula:

$$\log C_t = \frac{-k_e t}{2.303} + \log C_0$$

where C_t denotes the blood concentration of the drug at time t, k_e denotes the constant of clearance rate, and C_0 is the initial plasma concentration of the drug.

2. **Zero-order clearance kinetics**: This means that in vivo, the drug is cleared at a constant rate, namely, the amount of drug cleared within a unit time is consistent, irrespective of the drug concentration in the blood. The drug concentration-time curve that complies with zero-order clearance kinetics is presented as a straight line (Fig. 4.4), which is commonly the case when the clearance ability of the body has reached saturation. Zero-order clearance kinetics can be expressed using the following formula:

$$C_t = -k_0 t + C_0$$

where C_t denotes the blood concentration of the drug at time t, k_0 denotes the constant of zero-order clearance rate, and C_0 is the initial plasma concentration of the drug.

4.1.2 The Main Process of Pharmacokinetic Analysis in Clinical Pharmacology

The PK study of a drug always includes two parts, one is a preclinical PK study and the other one includes a clinical PK study, a bioavailability study, and a bioequivalence study. Before commencing the PK study, the study objective should be clearly defined, and a scientific and reasonable study design should be made depending on the specific characteristics and conditions of the drug. In traditional clinical pharmacology, a PK study always includes the following key steps: establishing a suitable method to assess the in vivo concentrations of the drug and testing it according to the study objective and the physical-chemical properties of samples waiting for analysis; conducting a compartment model fitting of the tested in vivo drug concentrations; calculating the basic kinetic parameters; and finally, instructing rational drug use in clinical practice, according to the rules of kinetic change of the drug deduced from the basic kinetic parameters.

4.1.2.1 In Vivo Measurement of the Drug Concentration

1. **Type, collection, and storage of biological samples**: The study objective and the physical-chemical properties of the drug determine the pattern of sample collection. The types of biological samples for in vivo drug analysis commonly include plasma, serum, whole blood, urine, saliva, and feces. In special conditions, the milk, tears, cerebrospinal fluid, bile, amniotic fluid, and even various tissues can be taken as biological samples for analysis. Rational setting of the time point of sample collection is critical to a PK study, which should cover the absorption phase, the distribution phase, and the clearance phase. Generally, 9–13 collection points should be arranged, including 2–3 points in the absorption phase, 2–3 points around the

peak concentration of the drug, 2–3 points in the distribution phase, and 4–6 points in the clearance phase. The whole time of sampling should cover a least 3–5 times the half-life of the drug, or at least continues to the time that the concentration of drug has decayed to 1/10 to 1/20 of its peak concentration. It is better to test and analyze the samples immediately after collection, to avoid degradation or other chemical changes of the target compound in the samples. However, in clinical practice, the collected samples are always stored via freezing and then thawed before testing.

2. **Pretreatment of biological samples before testing**: Whether the collected biological sample needs pretreatment (such as purification) or not depends on its impurities and the testing method used. When measuring the drug and its metabolites in vivo, pretreatment of the collected samples is needed in most conditions before testing, except in few cases in which the samples can be tested directly. The steps of sample pretreatment generally include: (1) Sample homogenization; (2) protein removal; (3) extraction of the drug and its metabolites from the samples; (4) enrichment of components to be tested in the samples; (5) derivatization of the components to be tested in the samples; and (6) if necessary, chemical modification of the components to be tested in the samples to establish better conditions for testing.
3. **Testing methods for biological samples**: Low drug concentrations mean that sensitive, accurate, and reliable methods are necessary to test the drug concentration in human biological samples (because of various impact factors and the limited amount of collected samples) for a better understanding of the in vivo kinetic characteristics in relation to drug absorption, distribution, and clearance. These methods mainly include: (1) Spectral analysis, including colorimetry, ultraviolet spectrophotometry, and fluorescence spectrophotometry; (2) chromatography, including thin-layer chromatography, gas chromatography, and high performance liquid chromatography; (3) high performance capillary electrophoresis; (4) immunoassays; (5) isotopic methods; and (6) bioassays. When selecting the method to analyze the drug in vivo, comprehensive attention should be paid to the structure, physio-chemical properties, the in vivo concentration of the drug, the amount of interference, the method used for drug pretreatment, the study conditions, and the study purpose.
4. **Validation of the analysis method of the biological samples**: To ensure its reliability, the testing method needs to be validated, including the following aspects: (1) Sensitivity, always expressed as limit of quantitation (LOQ). It is required that the method can test the concentration of drug after has cleared for 3–5 times its half-life or when its concentration has decreased to 1/10–1/20 of the C_{max}. (2) Specificity, which must be able to prove that the tested component is the prototype of the drug or its metabolites, considering that the impact of endogenous substances, related metabolites, or impurities can be excluded. (3) Precision, commonly expressed as the intra-day or inter-day coefficient of variation, in terms of relative standard deviation (RSD). An RSD <15% is required when performing concentration testing five times each at lower (close to LOQ), median, and upper level (close to upper limit) of the drug concentration within the range of the standard curve. Even around the LOQ concentration, an RSD <20% is required. (4) Accuracy (or the relative recovery rate), commonly expressed as the bias between tested concentrations and the real concentrations of quality control samples. Likewise, an RSD <15% is required when performing concentration testing five times each at the lower (close to LOQ), median, and upper level (close to upper limit) of the drug concentration within the range of the standard curve. Even around the LOQ concentration level, an RSD <20% is required. (5) Extraction recovery rate (also called the absolute recovery rate), which should also be validated at lower, median, and upper levels of the drug concentration, and the value should be larger than 50%. (6) Standard curve. A standard curve should be established for each biological sample, with at least five

data points for the drug concentration, covering the whole range of concentrations of the biological samples. Extrapolation is not allowed, the zero point cannot be included, and a correlation coefficient $r \geq 0.95$ is required. (7) Stability of the samples. For samples stored frozen, at room temperature, those requiring a freeze-thaw process, stability analysis is required. (8) Methodological quality control. Quality control is required during the testing of drug concentrations in biological samples. Blank, low, medium, and high concentration tubes must be designed, and a standard curve should be established.

5. **Study content**: The exact content is different between preclinical and clinical PK studies, both of which should be established according to the specific drug to be analyzed and the study purpose.

   The content of a preclinical PK study includes: (1) A blood drug concentration-time curve; (2) A tissue distribution test; (3) a plasma protein binding test; (4) an excretion test; (5) a structural transformation test; and (6) the effect on drug metabolism enzymes. For drugs that require multiple administrations, the PK study should be performed under conditions of both single and multiple administrations, and the difference in drug kinetics between these two conditions should be compared.

   The PK study content of a phase I clinical trial of a new drug that mainly based on healthy volunteers includes: (1) a PK study under conditions of single drug administration; (2) a PK study under conditions of multiple drug administration; and (3) the impact of food intake on the absorption of orally delivered drugs.

   The PK study content of phase II and phase III clinical trials of a new drug includes: (1) an in vivo PK study in patient or subjects, under conditions of both single and multiple drug administration; (2) a PK study of the new drug in relation to metabolic pathways and the structure of its metabolites; (3) a PK study regarding the interaction between the new drug and other drugs; and (4) PK studies in special populations, for example, the impact of impaired liver and kidney function, age, and race on drug kinetics.

   When performing a PK study, attention should be paid to the selection of experimental animal or subjects and the sample sizes; whether fasting is needed; the drug to analyze; the method of drug administration; the dosage; the food and drink consumed after drug administration; the setting of time points for sample collection; and the bioavailability and bioequivalence of the drug.

4.1.2.2 Compartment Model Chimerism

Before taking the tested concentrations of the drug in the blood or the urine for analysis to calculate the kinetic metrics, the appropriate compartment model should be selected. Common methods of selection include: (1) Graphing judgment; (2) judging through sum of squares of residuals; (3) judging through determining coefficients (R^2); (4) Akaike Information Criterion (AIC); and (5) F test. The exact content of these methods can be found in Pharmacology textbooks.

The selection of the model is associated with the study design and the method used to test the drug concentration. Different ways of drug administration and different testing methods requires different models. For the same data, different compartment models would result in significantly different kinetic parameters.

In real practice, the AIC method is commonly used to judge the suitability of a compartment model. If difficulty arises using the AIC method, the F test or the sum of squares of residuals could be used to aid the selection. Theoretically, compartment model analysis cannot handle too many compartments, which should be less than three.

4.1.2.3 Calculation of the Kinetic Parameters

When the compartment model is determined, the kinetic parameters of the drug are calculated using specific formulae, for example, the $T_{1/2}$, V_d, K_e, AUC, and CL for venous-injected drugs; the K_a, $T_{1/2}$, C_{max}, T_{max}, AUC, and F for non-venous-administered drugs; the absolute bioavailability for water-soluble drugs administered nonvenously, the time to peak concentration (T_{max}); and the steady-state peak concentration of sustained-release or controlled-release medications provided by the concentration-time curve when steady state has achieved after multiple administration. As mentioned above, if the suitability of the compartment model is difficult to judge or the drug is not suitable for analysis through any compartment model, if the time course of the drug in vivo complies with a linear process, the kinetic parameters can be analyzed through a non-compartment model. The exact content of these methods can be found in Pharmacology textbooks.

4.1.2.4 Considering the Dynamic Change Rules of a Drug In Vivo and Assessment of the Results

After the kinetic parameters have been obtained using the abovementioned methods, the next step is to use these parameters to consider the dynamic change rules of the drug in vivo, and to comprehensively analyze and assess the study results.

For a preclinical PK study, a comprehensive discussion regarding the in vivo pharmacokinetic characteristics of drug should be carried out, including characteristics related to drug absorption, distribution, metabolism, and clearance; the binding of the drug to plasma proteins; its accumulation level in the body and the main organs or tissues; and its excretion characteristics through the urine, feces, and bile.

For a clinical PK study, the in vivo dynamic changes of the drug in health volunteers and the impact of related diseases on pharmacokinetics of drug should be discussed, to reveal the influence of other medications on the tested drug and their interactions, to recognize the population-specific impact on drug pharmacokinetics, and to determine the relationship between blood concentration and the clinical pharmacological effect of the drug. Objective evaluation of the in vivo status of the drug also needs to be assessed, for example, its bioavailability and bioequivalence. Thereby, the kinetic parameters can be used to instruct the clinical use of drug, for example, calculating the initial dose, the maintenance dose, and the administration intervals, as well as formulating a medication plan for different administration routes. The relationship between the in vivo and ex vivo kinetic characteristics of a drug can be used to instruct the design and production of its preparations. In particular, the release rules of the drug can be revealed according to the concentration-time curve, which can be used to instruct the preparation of quick-, sustained-, and control-release medications.

4.1.3 Common Parameters in Clinical Pharmacology and Their Clinical Significance

The purpose of establishing a compartment model for fitting tested dynamic data is to acquire certain semiquantitative kinetic parameters that can characterize the distribution, metabolism, and excretion of drugs. This would facilitate the recognition of drug properties and finally instruct the utility of drug. The common kinetic parameters are introduced as follows:

4.1.3.1 Half-Life Time of Clearance

The half-life time of clearance ($T_{1/2}$) is the time by which the blood drug concentration decreases to a half of its initial concentration, which indicates the clearance rate of the drug. As mentioned above, most of the drugs comply with first-order-clearance kinetics, and thus have a constant $T_{1/2}$, which can be calculated through following formula:

$$T_{1/2} = 0.693 / k_e$$

where k_e is the constant of the clearance rate.

According to $T_{1/2}$, the intervals of drug administration can be determined. Generally, the longer the $T_{1/2}$, the larger intervals of drug administration, and vice versa. The interval of administration is always set at about one-fold of $T_{1/2}$. If the toxicity of the drug is low, the dose can be rationally increase, which reduces the frequency of drug administration and would ensure a substantial blood concentration of the drug within its administration interval. For drugs that are cleared via first-order kinetics, the in vivo amount of the drug would decrease to approximate 3%, after five times the $T_{1/2}$, indicating that the drug would have almost cleared from the body. Therefore, when the drug is administered at a constant dose and a constant interval, five times the $T_{1/2}$ later, the blood concentration of drug would achieve a steady state. From the $T_{1/2}$ of the drug, the time by which the steady-state blood concentration will be achieved under continuous administration and how long it will take for the drug to be almost completely cleared in vivo can be predicted.

For a drug that complies with first-order clearance kinetics, its half-life of clearance can be calculated as:

$$T_{1/2} = 0.5 \times \frac{C_0}{k_0}$$

For a drug that complies with zero-order clearance kinetics, its half-life of clearance is proportional to its concentration in blood, namely, the larger amount of drug administered, the longer of the $T_{1/2}$.

4.1.3.2 Clearance Rate

The clearance rate (CL) is defined as the plasma volume, in mL, from which the drug has cleared within a unit time. Thus, the CL is also called the plasma clearance rate. The CL is commonly expressed as volume in unit time (mL/min or L/h), and can be calculated using the following formula:

$$\mathrm{CL} = \frac{A}{\mathrm{AUC}_{0\to\infty}}$$

where A denotes the total amount of the drug, AUC is the integral of area under the drug concentration-time curve. For a drug that complies with first-order clearance kinetics, the proportion of the drug that clears within a unit time is a constant, and thus its CL is also a constant. When the clearance capacity has reached the saturation of the organic body, drug clearance will change to a zero-order-clearance pattern. At this time, the amount of drug cleared within a unit time is consistent, while the CL changes with time.

Under normal circumstances, the CL of the body is the sum of drug that is cleared by the liver, kidney, and other clearance organs, thus it is called the total CL. If it is only necessary to calculate the CL of a specific organ, then the nomenclature of organ-specific CL should be used, for example, liver CL ($\mathrm{CL}_{\mathrm{liver}}$) or kidney CL ($\mathrm{CL}_{\mathrm{kidney}}$), etc.

4.1.3.3 Bioavailability

Regardless of its administration method, the fraction of drug that has reached the blood circulation is defined as its bioavailability, F for short, which is calculated as follows:

$$F = \frac{A}{D} \times 100\%$$

where A is the total amount of the drug in vivo, while D is the drug dose.

Bioavailability reflects not only how much drug would enter the blood circulation of the body, but also its entry speed, as shown in Fig. 4.5. When administered with different dosage forms, the time to the maximum blood concentration of a drug reflects the speed difference of its bioavailability.

Bioavailability can be divided into relative and absolute bioavailability. Bioavailability is commonly calculated by comparing the amount of the drug in vivo; therefore, it is always expressed as the AUC of the blood drug concentration-time curve. The bioavailability of a venous-administered drug is considered to be 100%; therefore, when comparing the AUC of non-venous-administered drug with that of a venous-administered drug, absolute bioavailability is obtained. When comparing the AUC of a specific dosage form of a drug (for example, the same drug but in different dosage form produced by different companies) with those of its standard dosage form, the relative bioavailability is obtained.

4.1.3.4 Apparent Distribution Volume

When the distribution of a drug achieves equilibrium between the plasma and tissue, the "apparent" volume necessary to contain the entire amount of a drug is called the apparent volume of distribution (V_d), which can be expressed as:

$$V_{\mathrm{d}} = \frac{A}{C_0}$$

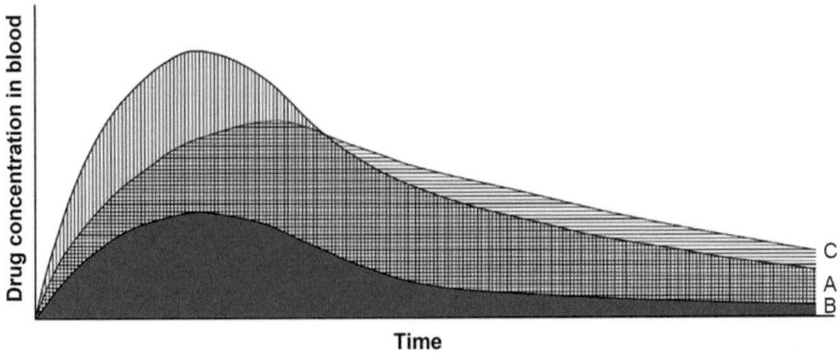

Fig. 4.5 Comparison of bioavailability among three different kinds of drugs. Drug A is absorbed quickly and completely. The absorption speed of drug B is similar to drug A, but dramatically less absorbed. Drug C is absorbed completely, but at a slower absorption speed than A

A is the total amount of drug in vivo, and C_0 is the plasma concentration of the drug when its distribution between the plasma and the tissue has achieved equilibrium.

As the drug is always distributed heterogeneously among different parts of the body, V_d is not a real volumetric space, but merely indicates the total fluid volume for distribution of the total in vivo drug when considering that the drug concentrations in all parts of the body are equal to the plasma concentration. Therefore, the distribution of the drug throughout the entire body can be estimated through V_d.

The significance of V_d lies in: (1) According to V_d, the total amount of the drug can be calculated for a given expected drug concentration. If the absorption fraction of drug is 100%, *A* equals the drug dosage. (2) According to V_d, the extent of drug distribution can be estimated. For example, if V_d is too large, drug accumulation in certain tissues or organs should be considered.

4.1.3.5 Maintenance Dose, Loading Dose, and Individualized Treatment

In most cases, multiple intermittent administrations of a drug are applied in clinics, aiming to keep the steady-state concentration (C_{ss}) within the range of the therapeutic concentration. Thus, it is necessary to calculate the maintenance dose. To maintain a specific plasma C_{ss} or a target concentration of a drug, adjustment to the speed of drug administration is required to make the speed of drug entry into, and clearance from, the body equal. The related formula is expressed as:

$$\text{Administration speed} = \frac{\text{CL} \times C_{SS}}{F} \text{ or } = \frac{\text{CL} \times \text{target concentration}}{F}$$

where CL denotes the drug clearance rate, *F* denotes the bioavailability, and C_{ss} denotes the steady-state concentration.

Administration speed is the ratio of dosage to administration interval, namely, the amount of the drug administered within a unit time interval. For a given ideal plasma concentration, clearance rate, and bioavailability of a drug, its dosage and administration interval can be calculated using the above formula.

When continuously given at a maintenance dosage, the C_{ss} of a drug can be achieved after 4–5 times the half-life. Neither increasing the dosage nor reducing the medication interval will make the C_{ss} arrive ahead of time. For patient that needs the C_{ss} to be achieved ahead of time to control the disease quickly, a loading dosage can be applied. A loading dosage means increasing the first dosage, and then giving the maintenance dosage continuously; this can make steady-state therapeutic concentration (or a target concentration set beforehand for the patient) occur ahead of time. The loading dosage can be calculated as:

$$\text{Loading dosage} = \frac{\text{target concentration} \times V_{SS}}{F}$$

where V_{ss} denotes the apparent distribution volume under the steady-state plasma concentration, and F denotes bioavailability.

In conclusion, to draw up a plan for drug administration, the F, CL, V_{ss}, and $T_{1/2}$ of drug must be obtained, and the absorption speed and distribution characteristics of the drug should be recognized. Based on the kinetic parameters of the drug, to design a reasonable drug administration plan always includes multiple steps, as follows: (1) select and determine the target concentration; (2) estimate the CL and V_d of the drug according to its PK parameters and the pathophysiological status of the patient (such liver and renal function); (3) calculate the loading dosage, maintenance dosage, and administration speed; (4) predict the time to C_{ss} according to the $T_{1/2}$ of the drug, and then test the C_{ss}; (5) calculate drug CL and V_d of the patient according to the tested C_{ss}; (6) adjust the target concentration of the drug according to the clinical requirements and the treatment response of the patient; and (7) rectify the target concentration of the drug and then start again from step three.

4.2 Pharmacokinetics in PET Imaging

Based on continuous PET dynamic imaging, the dynamic distribution of radioactive tracer in the body can be visualized, from which the kinetic information of the drug is implied. Acquiring information related to the clinical PK of a drug or even deeper information from the visualized continuous PET dynamic imaging, undoubtedly involves release pharmacokinetic analysis from traditional complex processes, and transforming into a pattern that is easier to operate with more connotations. To date, the analysis methods for the pharmacokinetics in PET imaging have been continuously improved.

4.2.1 Theoretical Introduction to Kinetic Modeling in PET

4.2.1.1 Compartment Model

Similar to related theories of PK in clinical pharmacology, the core concept of PK in PET imaging is also to consider the whole organic body system comprising multiple compartments. Compartments should not be understood as a physical volume, but rather as a mass of well-mixed, homogeneous material that behaves uniformly. Each compartment might exchange material with other compartments. Nuclear medicine applies tiny amounts of radioactive tracer; therefore, it is usually assumed that the observed system is not disturbed by the tracer. It is further assumed that the physiological conditions do not change during the study, such that the rate of material exchange can be considered as constant. There are obvious differences between PET kinetic modeling and PK in traditional clinical pharmacology, namely: (1) Kinetic modeling in PET only applies to drugs that are labeled with a radionuclide. (2) Kinetic modeling in PET only applies to that administered through a vein. (3) The meaning of compartments involved is different in these two kinetic methods. In compartment models of traditional clinical pharmacology, both drug administration and sampling are conducted through the central compartment. In contrast, in dynamic PET imaging, the time to activity curve (TAC) can be obtained from both the blood and from any tissue or organ by drawing a region of interest (ROI) in these areas, allowing for corresponding PK analysis. The key processes of PET kinetic modeling are illustrated in Fig. 4.6. (4) The relationship between different compartments in clinical pharmacology lies in material exchange and transfer between a central compartment with one or multiple peripheral compartments, which resembles a "paralleling" pattern. However, in PET kinetic modeling, compartments are divided mainly according to certain key steps (e.g., transmembrane transport and rate-limiting enzymes) in the pathway of drug

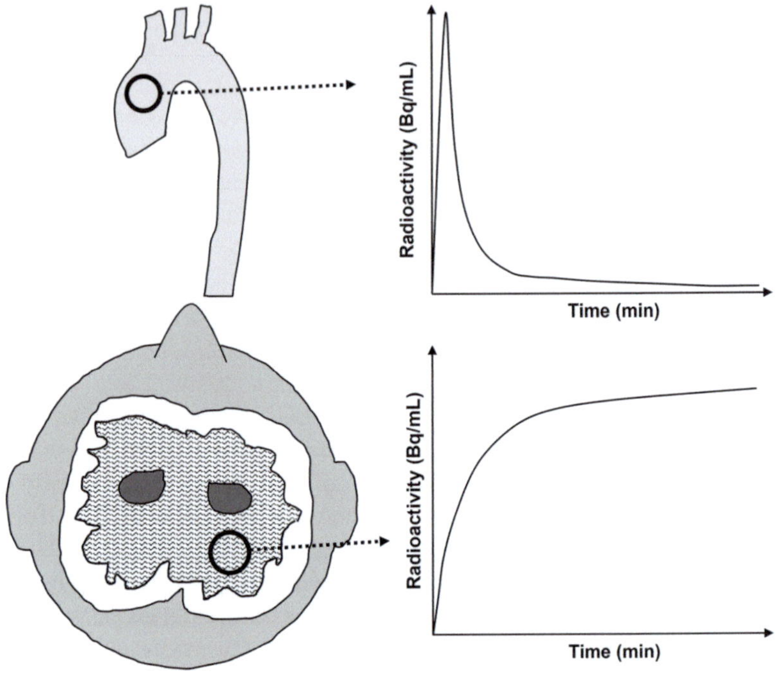

Fig. 4.6 Diagrammatic sketch illustrating ROI drawing and TAC generation

metabolism, resulting in different distribution rates in these compartments. Thus, this kind of relationship between different compartments tends to be a kind of "series connection." (5) In the PK of traditional clinical pharmacology, only one compartment model that is suitable for a specific drug can be used for analysis, e.g., a one compartment model or two compartment models. Nevertheless, in PET kinetic modeling, for drugs that are characterized by complex or high-level compartment model kinetics, simple or low-level compartment models can also be used to analyze the kinetic parameters of the drug, which depends on the specific study objectives, but only with a reduced number of parameters being obtained.

Similar to traditional clinical pharmacology, PET kinetic modeling also includes compartment models and non-compartment models, but with obviously different connotations.

1. **One tissue compartment model**: This is the simplest model, i.e., the drug is delivered quickly to the capillaries through the blood circulation and is transferred into specific tissues right after injection into the body. Some fraction of the tracer is extracted into tissue and metabolized, the rest is transported back to the blood, from where a new circulation starts, as shown in Fig. 4.7. Unlike the compartment model in clinical pharmacology, the one compartment model in PET kinetic modeling includes one blood-pool compartment and one tissue compartment, and thus is called a one tissue compartment model (1TCM).

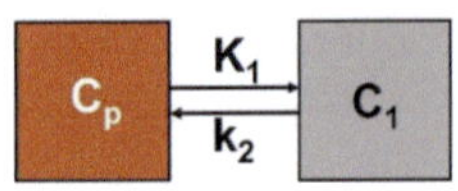

Fig. 4.7 Diagrammatic sketch of the 1-tissue-compartment model. C_p denotes the plasma concentration of the drug; C_1 denotes the drug concentration in tissue; K_1 and k_2 indicate the constant rates of drug delivery forward and backward from plasma to tissue, respectively

It is assumed that the arterial tracer concentration is the same throughout the body because of mixing, such that it can be measured in a peripheral artery, which is a prerequisite for using 1TCM. The tracer concentration in tissue $C_1(t)$ increases by the extraction of tracer from the arterial blood plasma, with a delivery rate in every moment proportional to the tracer concentration in plasma, and thus complies with first-order kinetics. A usual condition for quantitative analysis is that only the unchanged tracer, called the parent tracer, can enter tissue, whereas labeled metabolites, which may also circulate, cannot. Parallel to the uptake, tracer in tissue is reduced by a backward transfer (or washout), which is proportional to the concentration in tissue [$C_1(t)$]. Both processes compete, such that the change over time of the net tracer concentration in tissue ($\mathrm{d}C_1(t)/\mathrm{d}t$) can be expressed using the following differential equation:

$$\frac{\mathrm{d}C_1(t)}{\mathrm{d}t} = K_1 C_p(t) - k_2 C_1(t)$$

Attention should be paid to the two transfer coefficients, K_1 and k_2, which have somewhat different meanings, indicated by using capital and small letters. K_1 is commonly considered to have a relatively determined clinical significance, indicating a somewhat perfusion-dependent component of the tracer within a unit time, and thus units of milliliter per minute per cubic centimeter (mL/min/cm^3) are used. In PET kinetic modeling, a kinetic parameter that has a relatively clear clinical significance is commonly expressed in capital letters. In contrast, k_2 [min^{-1}] indicates the fraction of the drug transferred per unit time from tissue to blood. Generally, the plasma concentration $C_p(t)$ is not a compartment, but is considered as a measured quantity and appears as the input function that drives the system.

2. **Complex compartment model**

   In most cases, the drug will be carried to the next metabolic step or binds to a target receptor, and thus a more complex compartment model is required to better investigate the kinetic characteristics of the drug. Despite this, a basic three tissue compartment model (3TCM) is enough to characterize most drugs (Fig. 4.8). Namely, after entering a cell, the tracer is available for binding in a free form at a concentration $C_1(t)$. Free tracer can be directly bound to its target molecule or receptor, $C_2(t)$, but it also might bind to certain cell components or molecules that are not known in detail, $C_3(t)$. Considering these pathways, a 3TCM with six transfer coefficients (K_1, k_2, k_3, k_4, k_5 and k_6) was established, whereby C_2 and C_3 communicate only via C_1.

   The differential equations of 3TCM can be derived analogously to those of 1TCM, but are much more complex. The equations are expressed as follows:

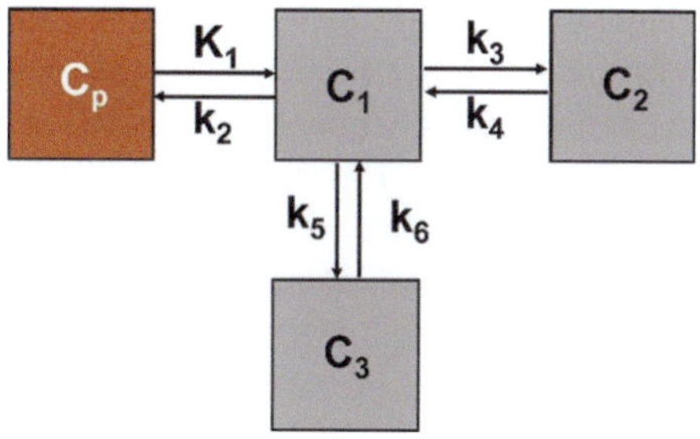

Fig. 4.8 Diagrammatic sketch of a 3-tissue-compartment model. C_p denotes the plasma concentration of the drug; C_1 denotes the drug concentration in tissue; K_1 and k_2 indicate the constant rates of drug delivery forward and backward from plasma to tissue, respectively; C_2 is the concentration of the drug that has bound to target molecules or receptors, with k_3 and k_4 indicating the corresponding transfer rates; C_3 is the concentration of the drug that has bound to certain cell components or molecules that are not known in detail, with k_5 and k_6 indicating corresponding transfer rates

$$\frac{\mathrm{d}C_1(t)}{\mathrm{d}t} = K_1 C_p(t) - (k_2 + k_3 + k_5) C_1(t) + k_4 C_2(t) + k_6 C_3(t)$$

$$\frac{\mathrm{d}C_2(t)}{\mathrm{d}t} = k_3 C_1(t) - k_4 C_2(t)$$

$$\frac{\mathrm{d}C_3(t)}{\mathrm{d}t} = k_5 C_1(t) - k_6 C_3(t)$$

3. **Two-tissue compartment model**

   Although the abovementioned 3TCM applies to most drugs, it contains six unknown parameters (K_1 to k_6) that are difficult to assess and calculate experimentally. Furthermore, the stabilities of the equations and results are difficult to guarantee. For practical purposes, the system is therefore most often reduced to a 2-tissue compartment model (2TCM) by treating free and non-specifically bound tracer as a single compartment C_1 (non-displaceable compartment), considering the small fraction and relative quick binding-releasing rate of the non-specifically bound tracer compared to specific binding. The process of 2TCM is illustrated in Fig. 4.9.

The differential equations of 2TCM are given by

$$\frac{dC_1(t)}{dt} = K_1 C_p(t) - (k_2 + k_3) C_1(t) + k_4 C_2(t)$$

$$\frac{dC_2(t)}{dt} = k_3 C_1(t) - k_4 C_2(t)$$

2TCM can be divided into reversible and irreversible 2TCM. If the binding rate is close to the release rate between the radioactive tracer and its target molecules or receptors, a reversible 2TCM is defined. If the binding rate is dramatically larger than the release rate, i.e., $k_3 \gg k_4$, an irreversible 2TCM should be established, as shown in Fig. 4.10.

Note that in dynamic PET imaging, the measured radioactive concentration of tissue $C_T(t)$ within a volume of interest (VOI) is the sum of all radioactive materials, including $C_1(t)$, $C_2(t)$, and the tracer concentration in the blood of the tissue. PET is unable to distinguish between $C_1(t)$ and $C_2(t)$.

If we use vB to represent the volume fraction of blood in tissue, and $C_B(t)$ to represent the tracer concentration of whole blood, then the measured radioactive concentration of tissue $C_T(t)$ can be calculated using following equation:

$$C_T(t) = (1 - vB) \times [C_1(t) + C_2(t)] + vB \times C_B(t)$$

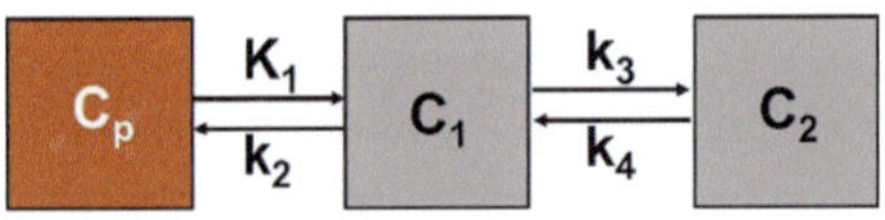

Fig. 4.9 Diagrammatic sketch of the reversible 2-tissue compartment model. C_p denotes the plasma concentration of the drug; C_1 denotes the drug concentration in tissue; K_1 and k_2 indicate the constant rates of drug delivery forward and backward from plasma to tissue, respectively; C_2 is the concentration of the drug that has bound to target molecules or receptors, with k_3 and k_4 indicating corresponding transfer rates

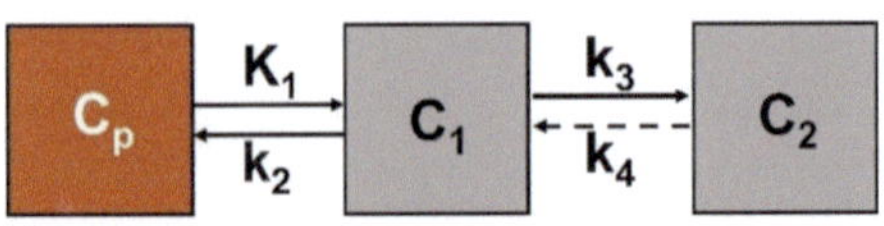

Fig. 4.10 Diagrammatic sketch of an irreversible 2-tissue compartment model. C_p denotes the plasma concentration of the drug; C_1 denotes the drug concentration in tissue; K_1 and k_2 indicate the constant rates of drug delivery forward and backward from plasma to tissue, respectively; C_2 is the concentration of the drug that has bound to target molecules or receptors, with k_3 and k_4 indicating the corresponding transfer rates, where $k_3 \gg k_4$

4.2.1.2 Non-compartment Models

The abovementioned models analyze TAC data through a non-linear regression pattern. Although this is the current standard method for PET kinetic modeling, it requires complex processing using mathematical algorithms. To this end, many methods that use a relatively simple process algorithm through linear regression are attracting increased attention. These methods are mostly used in graphic analysis or parametric imaging, with a relatively limited number of kinetic parameters that can be revealed. Herein, we introduce two mature and widely used methods that are based on linear regression.

1. **The Patlak Plot**

   The Patlak plot has been developed for systems with irreversible pharmacological kinetics. A typical case is its application for the analysis of ^{18}F-FDG, which can be modeled as a 2TCM with $k_4 = 0$. In the Patlak plot, the measured TAC undergoes a special transformation and is linear regressed against some sort of "normalized time". The measured PET activity is divided by plasma activity and plotted at a "normalized time" (integral of the input curve from injection divided by the instantaneous plasma activity). The equation of the Patlak plot is

$$\frac{C_T(t)}{C_P(t)} = K \frac{\int_0^t C_P(\tau)\,d\tau}{C_P(t)} + V$$

   This means that a Patlak plot will result in a straight line after sufficient equilibration time, as shown in Fig. 4.11. The slope and the

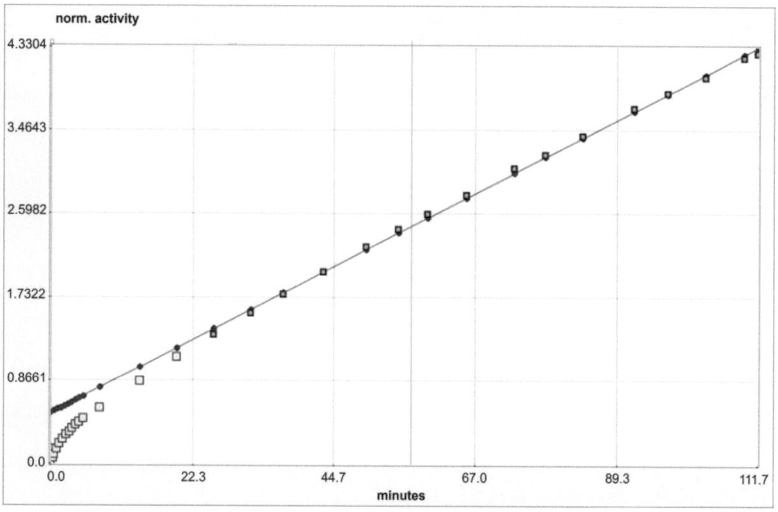

Fig. 4.11 Typical image illustrating Patlak plot fitting in PMOD software

intercept must be interpreted according to the underlying tracer and its compartment model kinetic characteristics. For ^{18}F-FDG, the slope K equals $K_1k_3/(k_2 + k_3)$ and represents the influx Ki, while the intercept V equals $V_0 + vB$ with the distribution volume V_0 of the reversible compartment C_1 and the fractional blood volume vB.

2. **Logan Plot**

   The Logan plot is another linear regression method developed for reversible 2TCM systems which allows estimating the total distribution volume V_t. The key concept of Logan plot is to perform a transformation to the measured TAC of the tissue $C_T(t)$, and then plot it at a "normalized time." The equation for Logan plot is

$$\frac{\int_0^t C_T(\tau)\mathrm{d}\tau}{C_T(t)} = K\frac{\int_0^t C_P(\tau)\mathrm{d}\tau}{C_T(t)} + b$$

   This means that the measured PET activity is integrated and divided by the instantaneous tissue activity and plotted at a "normalized time" (integral of input curve from injection divided by the instantaneous tissue activity). For suitable systems and after sufficient equilibration time, this plot will approach a straight line (Fig. 4.12). Like the Patlak plot, the kinetic metrics revealed by the Logan plot should also be interpreted according to the underlying tracer and its compartment model kinetic characteristics. The slope represents the total distribution volume V_t of the tracer (including the blood space), for the 1-tissue compartment model, $K=K_1/k_2 + vB=V_t$, for the 2-tissue compartment model, $K = K_1/k_2(1 + k_3/k_4 + vB) = V_t$.

   Note that both of the abovementioned two linear regression methods consider the contribution of blood activity to the total tissue activity, namely, the vB. Thus, correction should be performed to the measured activity of the tissue before the analysis as follows:

$$C_T(t) = \frac{C_{\mathrm{PET}}(t) - vB \times C_B(t)}{1 - vB}$$

Besides, as shown in Figs. 4.11 and 4.12, linear correlation cannot be achieved through the whole course of the data, between the transformed tissue activity concentration and the normalized time, neither in the Patlak plot nor in the Logan plot. An obvious deviation from the straight line can be visualized in the initial segments of the data. Thus, the data after a certain time (t^*) by which the steady state of tracer distribution has almost been achieved is commonly selected for analysis, where linear correlation is basically fulfilled. In particular, herein, the t^* was not a real time but the "normalized time."

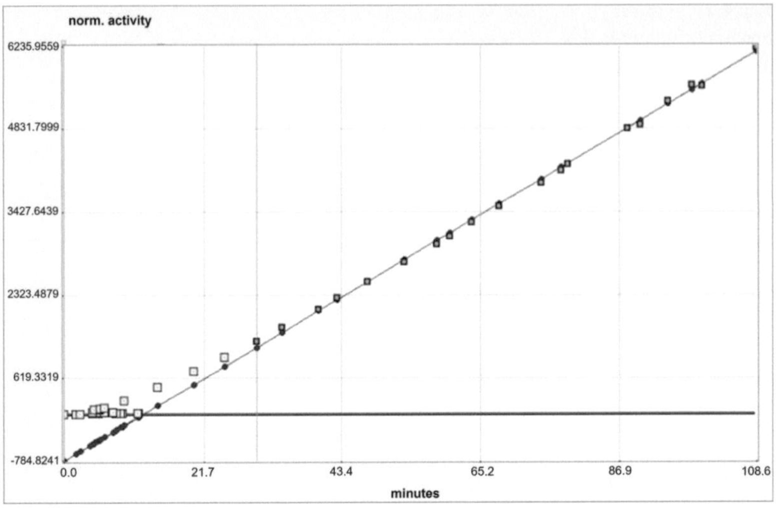

Fig. 4.12 Typical image illustrating Logan plot fitting in PMOD software

4.2.2 Main Steps of Pharmacokinetic Analysis in PET

As mentioned above, two sets of TAC data must be obtained before the PK analysis of the tracer, either in compartment model or in non-compartment model analysis, namely, the arterial plasma TAC data and the tissue TAC data, expressed as $C_P(t)$ and $C_T(t)$, respectively, with the former commonly used as the input function. Then, model fitting is performed using compartment or non-compartment models to obtain basic kinetic constant rates, such as K_1, k_2, k_3, k_4, and vB, through certain specific non-linear or linear functions. These basic constant rates are commonly called the micro kinetic parameters of the drug, which can be further used to calculate the macro kinetic parameters of drug, such as Ki, V_t, Vs, and V_{ND}, according to the PK characteristics of the drug. Finally, the kinetic characteristics of a drug can be assessed using these micro and macro kinetic parameters; these are the main steps of PK analysis in PET.

4.2.2.1 Input Function

When a radioactive tracer enters the blood circulation, not all of it can be extracted by tissue freely. The whole blood of an organic body always comprises blood cells (including red blood cells and white blood cells) and plasma. The tracer in the whole blood includes its free state distributed in blood cells and in the plasma, the combined state that is bound to specific plasma proteins, and its plasma metabolites, all of which contribute to the emission component of the radioactive tracer. However, only the free and parent state of tracer can be extracted by tissue, and thus can be used as the input curve in model fitting. Thus, direct or indirect methods are needed to separate each component of the radioactive tracer in the whole blood, to obtain the plasma TAC [$C_P(t)$], for use as the input function in model fitting.

1. **Arterial blood sampling**:

   After the injection of the tracer, continuous invasive collection of arterial blood samples is the standard method to obtain an input curve. To do this, the following blood analysis steps are required: First, separation of the plasma from the blood cells by centrifugation. Second, further separation of tracer in the plasma into tracer metabolites and unchanged tracer by filtration or high performance liquid chromatography (HPLC), to obtain the free and unchanged concentration of the tracer, also called the parent concentration. Generally in this step, only the instantaneous fraction of the parent concentration (the value ranges from 0 to 1) can be obtained, which can be multiplied by $C_p(t)$ to get the input function, as shown in Fig. 4.13. Although the tracer concentration in a peripheral artery can be taken as equal to that in a central large artery,

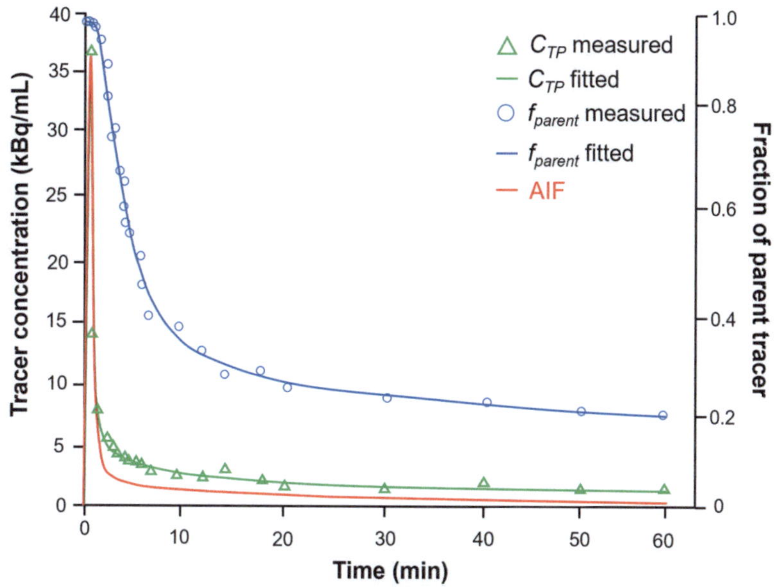

Fig. 4.13 Image illustrating how the arterial input function (AIF) obtained from the measured total plasma concentration of the tracer (C_{TP})

blood sample collections by continuous invasive punctures to the peripheral artery is not practical. In the first place, it is unacceptable for the subjects, in the second place, it is unable to capture the early kinetic information of the tracer, which requires the collection of a blood sample within a couple of seconds. Thus, the most practical method is the puncture and catheterization of the central large artery, and continuously collecting blood samples through an extended catheter.

2. **Image-derived input function**

   It is obvious that the abovementioned invasive method for obtaining the arterial input function (AIF) is complex and unsuitable for clinical practice. For some tracers that are characterized by ligand-receptor binding kinetics, the whole blood time-to-activity curve $C_B(t)$ can used, instead of $C_P(t)$, as the input function, measured through drawing a VOI in the central large artery, if the stability of tracer can be guaranteed with the time of dynamic PET imaging and no target receptor is expressed on the membrane of blood cells. This purely image-derived input function (IDIF) is increasingly used in clinics.

3. **Image and blood sampling combined input function**

   A compromise method is to obtain the input function through a combination of blood sampling and IDIF. Namely, 5–7 blood samples were collected from peripheral veins during dynamic PET imaging. Then, separation of the plasma from the blood cells by centrifugation is conducted, and a fraction of the plasma is obtained for each sample, from which the average fraction is used for correction of IDIF (multiplying the average fraction by the IDIF) to get the corrected image-derived input function (cIDIF) [5]. Compared with the IDIF, cIDIF is considered as closer to the real AIF. However, this method neglects the phenomenon by which the fraction of tracer distribution between blood cells and plasma changes dramatically over time during dynamic PET scanning.

4.2.2.2 Dynamic PET Imaging, Image Reconstruction, and TAC Generation

Before PET kinetic modeling, the second data that should be obtained is the tracer activity-to-time curve, namely, $C_T(t)$, which can be measured through VOI drawing on dynamic PET images, described as follows:

1. **Dynamic PET imaging and image reconstruction**

   When performing injection of the radioactive tracer, it is better to choose a large vein and conduct in a bolus injection; this is helpful to obtain a good IDIF. Start the dynamic PET scanning simultaneously after the injection of the radioactive tracer. Thanks to the dramatically improved spatial and temporal resolution of the uEXPLORER total-body PET/CT scanner, continuous dynamic PET imaging is allowed. To capture substantial kinetic information for the tracer, an acquisition time of more than 60 min is commonly required. However, it is reported that the acquisition time of dynamic PET could be reduced to 45 min [6] or even to 30 min [7]. The images are corrected for radioactive decay, attenuation, scatter, and randoms and are reconstructed using the list-mode ordered-subsets expectation-maximization algorithm incorporating TOF and point spread function modeling (OSEM-TOF-PSF). Then, the images are divided into a series of frames: every 5 s a frame for the initial 3 min (36 × 5 s) and every 3 min a frame thereafter until the end (24 × 180 s).

2. **VOI delineation in tissue and TAC generation**

   The VOI delineation depends on the specific tracer awaiting analysis and the corresponding study objectives. Considering the irregular shapes and non-homogeneous components of most organs, it is impractical to delineate the VOI of the entire organ. Therefore, for the purpose of analyzing the distribution of the tracer in normal organs, it is recommended to delineate multiple VOIs in different areas within the organ, which would result in multiple TAC data and multiple values of the kinetic parameters after model fitting, then the average value is taken to represent the entire kinetic characteristics of the organ. If the purpose is to analyze the kinetic characteristics of the tracer in lesions, it is recommended to use the threshold segmentation method for VOI delineation, which would reduce operator bias. For example, the automatically adaptive segmentation method or the segmentation method using an isocontour threshold of 40% SUV_{max} can be regarded as a good method [8], as shown in Fig. 4.14. Each VOI will generate a data set of TAC, in which the mean value of the radioactive concentration is recommended to be used to obtain a stable model fitting and the corresponding kinetic parameters.

4.2.2.3 Model Fitting and Parameter Generation

1. **Model fitting to the input curve**

   The limited sampling times, which are not available to match each frame of the dynamic PET images (actually not necessary), and the various impact factors that always result in substantial statistical variance of the sample data, mean that it is necessary to perform model fitting of the collected data of the input curve, before loading into PMOD software for model fitting of TAC data in tissue. For the fitted model curve, values that are missing from collected data of the input curve at any frame time of the dynamic PET images can be interpolated, leading to a complete input curve used for model fitting of tissue. The model recommended for fitting of the input curve is the 3-exponential function, as shown in Fig. 4.13.

2. **Model fitting to the TAC of tissue and the generation of kinetic parameters**

   When both the input curve and the tissue TAC are ready, the next step is to perform model fitting to the tissue TAC data. Considering that typical compartment model fitting is still the standard method to analyze PK characteristics of radioactive tracers, it is recommended to use the Kinetic module of PMOD for kinetic modeling, as shown in Fig. 4.15. According to the predicted kinetic characteristics (based on previous references or preclinical data) of the tracer awaiting analysis and the main study objectives, a suitable model can be selected based on the following principles: (1) It is recommended to start model fitting from simple models to complex models, for example from 1TCM to 2TCM, and then to 3TCM, if necessary. (2) There is no good or bad for model itself; however, if it can match the measured TAC data as much as possible, then the model is good. Thus, it is better try several models when performing model fitting, and select the best model for use after comparing its goodness of fit. (3) Theoretically, the higher the number of constants enrolled for fitting, the better goodness-

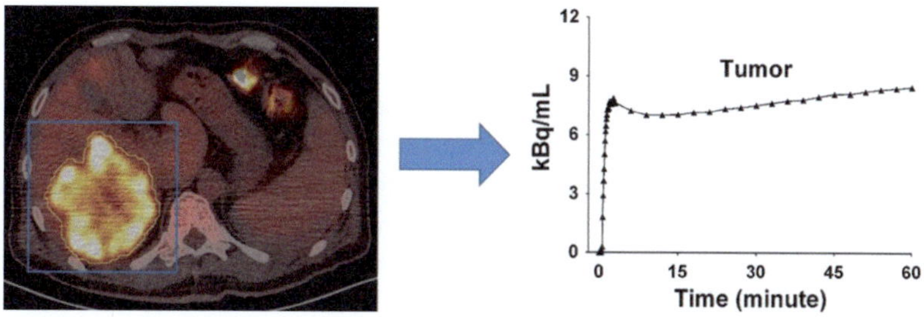

Fig. 4.14 Typical case illustrating VOI delineation around a hepatic tumor through the automatically adaptive segmentation method and the generation of TAC data

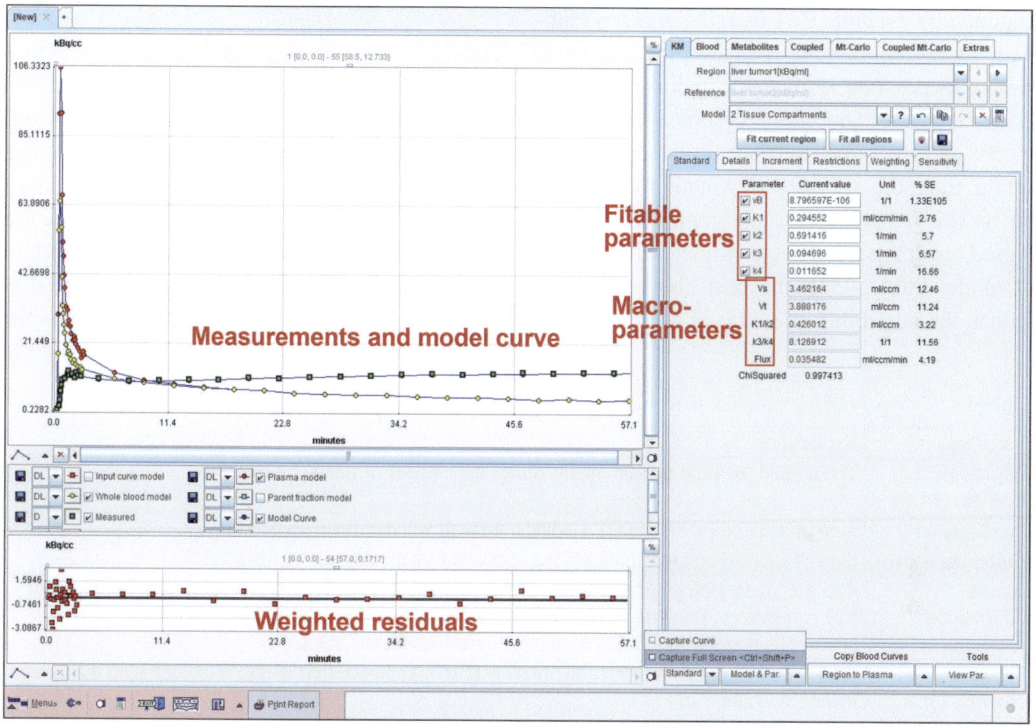

Fig. 4.15 Typical case illustrating mode fitting to tissue TAC data

of-fit will bet, if it can be calculated using the PMOD software. (4) As shown in Fig. 4.15, to reduce the spillover effect from radioactivity in blood cells to the measured plasma radioactivity, it is required to load both the whole TAC data and the plasma TAC data when perform model fitting.

4.2.2.4 Parametric Imaging

With the improvement of techniques in PET dynamic imaging, pixel-wise parametric calculation is becoming available through certain linear regression models (e.g., the Patlak plot and the Logan plot, etc.), resulting in parametric imaging of a specific kinetic parameter (such as *Ki*). With the advent of long-axial-FOV, the detection sensitivity and the temporal resolution of PET scanners has improved dramatically, and thus even a pixel-wise parametric calculation based on compartment model algorithms has become possible in clinics, leading to as many parametric images as is desired, such as K_1, k_2, k_3, and k_4 images. Based on these parametric images, kinetic metrics can be directly measured by drawing an ROI or VOI in these images, thus avoiding the complex process of compartmental model fitting. More importantly, these parametric images provide a visual image of a specific kinetic parameter of the tracer, which would facilitate precise and accurate diagnosis and disease therapy according these kinetic parametric images.

4.2.2.5 Evaluation of the Goodness of Model Fitting

Theoretically speaking, if it can match the measured TAC data as much as possible, the model is good. Commonly, the physiological behavior of drug is complicated, always needing complex compartment models with many constant rates included for model fitting to better characterize the kinetic features of a drug. However, the signal captured by dynamic PET imaging is always limited, which requires the selected model to be as simple as possible and cannot include too many constant rates. The more complex a selected model and the more constant rates included for fitting, the more accurate the kinetic metrics will be; however, this involves a larger possibility of a biased result arising. The assessment of goodness of model fitting seeks the best choice that can reduce the possibility of a biased result as much as possible without compromising any reliability of the results. There are many statistical variables that can be used to assist evaluation of goodness of model fitting, as listed in Table 4.1.

4.2.3 Common Parameters in PET Kinetic Modeling and Their Clinical Significance

The PK parameters of PET kinetic modeling include micro- and macroparameters. Microparameters can be obtained directly from compartment modeling and represent the basic delivery rate between compartments, including K_1, k_2, k_3, k_4, and vB. Except for K_1 and vB, the exact clinical significance of these parameters remains unclear and varies according to the different drugs analyzed. The macroparameters can

Table 4.1 Summary of the variables in relation to goodness of model fitting

Variables	Explanation
Degree of freedom (DOF)	The number of valid measurements minus the number of fitted parameters
SumSquared	Sum of squared (unweighted) residuals. A small value indicates a good fit
ChiSquared test	Sum of squared and weighted residuals, divided by the degrees of freedom
Akaike information criterion (AIC)	The AIC methodology attempts to find the model that best explains the data with a minimum of free parameters. The AIC is calculated with the second order correction for small sample size (<40). The preferred model is the one with the lowest AIC value
Schwartz criterion (SC)	Also called Bayesian information criterion (BIC). The preferred model is the one with the lowest SC value
Model selection criterion (MSC)	A criterion used in the scientist software to assess goodness of fitting. The preferred model is the one with the highest MSC value
R^2	Also called the coefficient of determination. R^2 is a common statistical variable used to assess the goodness of fit, with the value ranging between 0 and 1. A value of 0 means that the fit is not better than a horizontal line through the mean of all measurements, whereas a value of 1 means that all measurements lie exactly on the curve. High R^2 values indicate that the model curve is close to the measurement
Sy.x	This is defined as the standard deviation of the residuals and can be used to generate synthetic measurements in Monte Carlo simulations, provided all measurements have the same variability. The preferred model is the one with the lowest Sy.x value
Run test	The runs test is a statistical test to decide whether the model curve deviates systematically from the data. It is based on the number of runs resulting from the fit. A run is a set of consecutive measurements which are above (positive residuals) or below (negative residuals) the measurement. Given the assumption that the residuals are randomly distributed, the probability p of the occurrence of a number of runs can be calculated. If p is small (e.g., $p < 0.05$), the measurements systematically deviate from the model curve. Such a finding signals that an inadequate model was most likely fitted and further investigations of the result are not sensible. A value of 1 indicates a systematic deviation between the model and measurement ($p < 0.05$). A value of 0 means there is no significant deviation (https://doc36.pmod.com/pkin/4003.htm)
Area under curve (AUC)	Area under the model curve

not be acquired directly through compartment modeling but are commonly calculated from the micro parameters or from non-compartment modeling. In contrast to microparameters, macroparameters always have a clear clinical meaning, such as Ki, V_t, V_s, and V_{ND}.

4.2.3.1 Micro Kinetic Parameters

1. K_1: K_1 is the constant rate of drug delivery from plasma to tissue, with the unit of mL/(min cm^3). As mentioned earlier, K_1 is related to bioavailability F, expressed as:

$$K_1 = E \times F$$

where E represents the unidirectional first-pass extraction fraction (i.e., the fraction of the tracer that penetrates the capillary wall and is extracted into the tissue during the first pass of tracer through the capillary). The reverse transport is not regarded in the calculation of E, because drug concentration in tissue currently is zero. The extraction E can be calculated as:

$$E = 1 - \mathrm{e}^{-PS/F}$$

where P denotes the permeability, and S, the surface of the endothelium by which the capillary exchanges with the tissue. This relation demonstrates that if the permeability P of the capillary is large enough such that that it is dramatically higher than F, the extraction is virtually independent of F, and E approaches 1. Therefore, for tracers with high permeability, such as $^{15}O\text{-}H_2O$ and $^{13}N\text{-}NH_3$, K_1 is equal to F. In this case, K_1 can be obtained through fitting 1TCM of the tracer, and can be used to assess the blood perfusion of tissue.
2. k_2: k_2 represents the fractional rate constant for the washout of free tracer from tissue to plasma, with a unit of min^{-1}. It is a composite rate constant with unclear clinical significance; however, it is related to flow in the same way as K_1. Consequently, it is often reasonable to assume that the ratio K_1/k_2 is insensitive to flow and indicates a constant rate that is associated with the net influx of tissue.
3. k_3: k_3 occurs in 2TCM fitting and is regarded as the association rate of the ligand with specific binding sites (target molecules or receptors) or the rate of key rate-limiting enzymes that metabolize the tracer; it has a unit of min^{-1}. It is hard to find any kinetic feature of drug that is directly associated with k_3; however, it is a function of the concentration of the free radioligand, the available binding sites, and intrinsic second order association rate constants. Consequently, it is the foundation to assess the binding potential of the drug to specific sites.
4. k_4: k_4 is a basic constant rate of reversible 2TCM and is considered as the dissociation rate constant of the receptor–ligand complex, with a unit of min^{-1}. k_4 indicates, to some extent, the retention time of the tracer in tissue. In addition, similar to k_3, k_4 is also the foundation rate for assessing the binding potential of the drug to specific sites.
5. vB: vB represent the blood fraction in tissue, which is commonly used as a basic parameter in modeling of tissue TAC but is rarely used to assess the kinetic features of the drug. However, it has been reported that vB exhibits important additional values in tumor diagnosis, grading, staging, and gene expression prediction [9–11].

4.2.3.2 Macro Kinetic Parameters

Compared with the micro parameters, macro kinetic parameters are commonly calculated from a group of micro parameters, and thus are more indicative of certain kinetic features of the tracer. There are many parameters of this kind, with varying meanings depending on the tracer analyzed and the model used, of which some commonly used macro parameters are listed below.

1. Ki: also called metabolic influx, which indicates the overall rate at which the tracer is delivered from the blood to tissue, taken up, and then retained by the cells in the 2TCM system. It has a unit of mL/min/cm^3, and can be calculated as:

$$Ki = \frac{K_1 \times k_3}{k_2 + k_3}$$

The direct clinical significance of Ki is that it can be used to assess the metabolic rate of the tracer in tissue when multiplied with the plasma concentration of the tracer. Taking ^{18}F-FDG as an example, its metabolic rate in tissue can be calculated as follows:

$$\mathrm{MR}_{\mathrm{FDG}} = \mathrm{CGlu}_{\mathrm{P}} \times \frac{K_1 \times k_3}{k_2 + k_3}$$

where $\mathrm{MR}_{\mathrm{FDG}}$ denotes metabolic rate of ^{18}F-FDG, and $\mathrm{CGlu}_{\mathrm{P}}$ is the plasma concentration of glucose. $\mathrm{MR}_{\mathrm{FDG}}$ can be used further to calculate the metabolic rate of glucose in tissue as follows:

$$\mathrm{MR}_{\mathrm{Glu}} = \frac{\mathrm{CGlu}_{\mathrm{P}}}{\mathrm{LC}} \times \frac{K_1 \times k_3}{k_2 + k_3}$$

where LC (lumped constant) is a constant that indicates the difference of metabolism between ^{18}F-FDG and glucose in tissue. Different tissues might have different LCs. For example, the LC was reported to be 0.67 [12] and 1.2 [13] in the myocardium and skeletal muscle, respectively.

2. V_{S}: namely the distribution volume of specific binding, which is defined by the ratio of the specific binding concentration to the total parent concentration at equilibrium (which might not occur during the experiment). V_{S} is commonly used to assess the total amount of ligand–receptor drug binding to the specific sites. In 2TCM and 3TCM systems, V_{S} can be calculated as:

$$V_{\mathrm{S}} = \frac{K_1}{k_2} \times \frac{k_3}{k_4}$$

3. V_{T}: namely the total distribution volume, with a unit of mL/cm^3. If the assumption of rapid equilibration is not justified, one must resort to considering the entire tracer concentration in tissue as an indicator of specific binding, instead of V_{S}. The measure used in these cases is called the "total distribution volume" V_{T}, which is defined as the ratio of the tracer concentration in tissue to the total parent concentration in plasma at equilibrium. The clinical significance of V_{T} approximates to that of the apparent distribution volume in clinical pharmacology. For example, V_{T} can be a useful measure to guide the dosing of receptor targeted cancer drugs [14]. The calculation formula of V_{T} differs between 1TCM and 2TCM as follows:

$$V_{\mathrm{T}} = K_1 / k_2 \quad \text{1TCM}$$

$$V_{\mathrm{T}} = K_1 / k_2 \left(1 + k_3 / k_4\right) \quad \text{2TCM}$$

4. V_{ND}: namely the non-displaceable distribution volume, which can be interpreted in a ligand–receptor 2TCM system as the distribution volume of free and non-specifically bound tracer in the first compartment (C_1). This naming originates from the phenomenon that the concentration of free and non-specifically bound tracer in tissue is not reduced when a non-labeled ligand is brought into the tissue, competing with binding to the same receptor as the tracer. The rationale for this assumption is that the potential for non-specific binding to various cell components is practically unlimited as compared to the number of specific binding sites. V_{ND} can be calculated as:

$$V_{\mathrm{ND}} = K_1 / k_2 \quad \text{2TCM}$$

5. BP: namely the binding potential, which in ligand–receptor 2TCM systems, quantifies the equilibrium concentration of specific binding as a ratio to some other reference concentration. In particular, the ratio at equilibrium of a specifically bound radioligand to that of the non-displaceable radioligand in tissue is referred to as $\mathrm{BP}_{\mathrm{ND}}$ (unitless), which calculated as:

$$\mathrm{BP}_{\mathrm{ND}} = k_3 / k_4$$

4.3 Typical Cases Illustrating Tracer Distribution Analysis Through Total-Body PET/CT

Limited by the axial field of view (AFOV) of traditional PET/CT (15–30 cm), dynamic PET imaging is restricted to one bed position. In recent years, the multiple-bed multiple-pass imaging protocol has been proposed for whole-body dynamic PET imaging using traditional

PET/CT scanners; however, its temporal resolution is limited, and is thus incapable of capturing early kinetic features of the tracer, especially those with a fast metabolism [15, 16]. Furthermore, the parametric imaging based on this imaging protocol always has a low image signal-to-noise ratio [15, 16]. With the advent of long-AFOV PET/CT scanners, simultaneous total-body dynamic PET imaging within "one bed position" becomes possible, with a dramatically improved temporal resolution and signal-to-noise ratio, thanks to the >40-fold increase in detection sensitivity. These advantages of long-AFOV PET/CT scanner in dynamic PET imaging paved the way for analyzing the kinetic correlations between remote organs in the future, for example the brain–gut axis and the brain–heart axis. The authors believe that any new radioactive tracer should undergo total-body dynamic PET imaging using the long-AFOV PET/CT scanner to investigate its pharmacological characteristics before putting to clinical use. The simultaneous investigation of kinetic metrics of new tracers among multiple systems and multiple organs would serve as a "gold standard" reference for disease diagnosis. Based on our previous study results, herein, we introduce the kinetic distribution features in normal organs of three commonly used radioactive tracers.

4.3.1 Total-Body Dynamic PET Imaging to Investigate the Kinetic Distribution Features of ^{18}F-FDG in Normal Organs

^{18}F-FDG was called the century molecule, given its great contribution as a PET tracer to assess various pathologies. The kinetic features of ^{18}F-FDG have always been a concern. Some previous dynamic studies were based on an input function obtained from arterial blood sampling. Although the investigated results would be much closer to the "truth value," the invasive method used for artery blood sampling is not suitable for widespread clinical application. In contrast, the kinetic metrics of ^{18}F-FDG obtained through PET imaging would serve as a direct reference for its widespread application in clinics, although with certain bias to the "truth value."

To do this, the authors enrolled nine healthy volunteers for study [17]. Total-body dynamic PET imaging for 75 min was performed in these subjects using the long-AFOV uEXPLORER scanner. The dynamic PET data were reconstructed and divided into 60 frames: a frame every 5 s for the initial 3 min (36 × 5 s) and a frame every 3 min thereafter until the end (24 × 180 s). Then, ROIs were drawn within the organ boundary in the cerebral cortex, the cerebral white matter, the cerebellum cortex, the thyroid, the myocardium, the lung, the ascending aorta artery, the liver, the spleen, the pancreas, the kidney, the skeletal muscle, the bone, and the bone marrow, to obtain the TAC data of these tissues. Considering that obvious clearance of ^{18}F-FDG could be seen within 75 min of dynamic imaging, a reversible 2TCM was adopted for model fitting, as shown in Fig. 4.16. In this compartment model, the constant rates indicated the transport of ^{18}F-FDG forward (K_1) and backward (k_2) from plasma to tissue, and ^{18}F-FDG phosphorylation (k_3), and dephosphorylation (k_4). Finally, model fitting to tissue TAC data was performed, taking the TAC data from ascending aorta artery as the input function. The results for the kinetic metrics are summarized in Table 4.2.

As given in Table 4.2, the constant rates varied to a great degree among the organs. In most of the organs, the k_2 constants were much larger than the K_l constants, potentially indicating a major role of ^{18}F-FDG clearance during the time course. The exceptional organ was the liver, in which k_2 (0.5089 ± 0.0793) was relatively close to k_1 (0.4134 ± 0.0473), indicating that the ^{18}F-FDG metabolism of the normal liver might remain stable for a long time. Cluster analyses through iterative partitioning with the maximum likelihood criteria were performed to identify organs with similar kinetic characteristics; the results are given in Fig. 4.17.

As given in Fig. 4.17, an optimum of four groups of organs was obtained. The first group had the lowest K_l and k_3 and consisted of the white matter of the brain, the lung, the liver, the

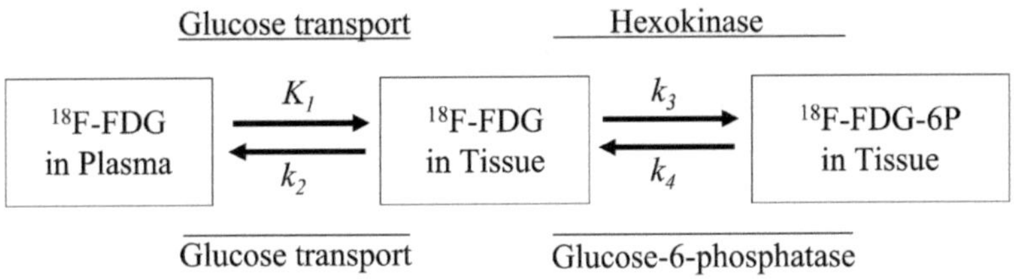

Fig. 4.16 Schematic diagram of the ^{18}F-FDG two-tissue compartment kinetic model

Table 4.2 Summary statistics of the kinetic metrics of ^{18}F-FDG in normal organs

Organs	K_1 (mL/min/cm^3)	k_2 (min^{-1})	k_3 (min^{-1})	MR_{FDG} (μmol/100 g/min)
Cerebral cortex	0.0896 ± 0.0225	0.2532 ± 0.1626	0.2213 ± 0.1190	23.1696 ± 3.3054
White matter	0.0337 ± 0.0080	0.1347 ± 0.0455	0.0482 ± 0.0151	7.6003 ± 1.5807
Cerebellum	0.1318 ± 0.0716	0.6280 ± 0.3728	0.1870 ± 0.1103	22.2233 ± 2.7109
Thyroid	0.9663 ± 0.3436	4.6042 ± 1.9598	0.0748 ± 0.0317	10.6186 ± 5.3299
Myocardium	0.8162 ± 0.5912	3.4975 ± 2.240	0.1909 ± 0.1013	17.9395 ± 13.4310
Lung	0.0143 ± 0.0083	0.3628 ± 0.2387	0.0307 ± 0.0240	0.5945 ± 0.4170
Liver	0.4134 ± 0.0473	0.5089 ± 0.0793	0.0129 ± 0.0065	5.224 ± 2.6668
Spleen	0.8846 ± 0.2058	2.0169 ± 0.4931	0.0415 ± 0.0245	9.4001 ± 4.5722
Pancreas	0.3561 ± 0.1496	1.7077 ± 0.4647	0.0787 ± 0.0336	8.2122 ± 4.0378
Kidney	0.7023 ± 0.1919	1.3542 ± 0.5321	0.1778 ± 0.1376	9.1456 ± 6.4375
Muscle	0.0263 ± 0.0156	0.3165 ± 0.1538	0.0461 ± 0.0263	1.8139 ± 0.7345
Bone	0.1544 ± 0.0484	0.7132 ± 0.2577	0.0458 ± 0.0151	4.997 ± 1.1549
Bone marrow	0.0405 ± 0.0134	0.2901 ± 0.0898	0.0189 ± 0.0054	1.3437 ± 0.4579

This table was adapted with permission from a published EJNMMI article [17]

Groups	Organs	K_1 (mL/min/cm^3)	k_2 (min^{-1})	k_3 (min^{-1})
1	Cerebral cortex Cerebellum	0.1107	0.3406	0.2041
2	Thyroid Myocardium	0.8912	4.0508	0.1329
3	Spleen Pancreas Kidney	0.6477	1.6929	0.0993
4	White matter Lung Liver Muscle Bone Bone marrow	0.0971	0.3709	0.0339

Fig. 4.17 Mean constant rates of organs with close kinetic metrics revealed using cluster analysis. (This figure was adapted with permission from a published EJNMMI article [17])

muscle, the bone, and the bone marrow, representing a low level of metabolism; another group demonstrated K_i values similar to those of the organs from group 1, but with the lowest k_2 and the highest k_3, indicating high avidity for FDG, and consisted of the cerebral and cerebellar cortices. A third group included the LV myocardium and the thyroid, which had the highest K_i and k_2, but a relatively lower k_3, indicating rapid metabolism but low utilization of FDG; the last group, consisting of the pancreas, the spleen, and the kidney, was distinguished from the third group mainly by somewhat lower values of K_i and k_3.

4.3.2 Total-Body Dynamic PET Imaging in Investigating Kinetic Distribution Features of ^{68}Ga-DOTA-TATE in Normal Organs

There is a unique advantage of somatostatin receptor (SSTR)-targeting PET imaging in the diagnosis of neuroendocrine tumors (NETs). It has demonstrated significant instructive values in diagnosis, staging, and treatment-strategy establishment of patients with NET. Of the various tracers synthesized, ^{68}Ga-DOTA-TATE has shown excellent affinity to SSTR, and thus has been widely used in clinics, which also represents the first ^{68}Ga-labeled SSTR analog to obtain approval from the US FDA. However, no study has reported the systemic kinetic metrics of ^{68}Ga-DOTA-TATE in normal organs.

Recently, the authors retrospectively enrolled seven patients who had received total-body ^{68}Ga-DOTA-TATE dynamic PET imaging, but with non ^{68}Ga-DOTA-TATE avid lesions identified on PET images [18]. All patients underwent 60-min total-body dynamic PET imaging using the long-AFOV uEXPLORER scanner. The dynamic PET data were reconstructed and divided into 55 frames: a frame every 5 s for the initial 3 min (36 × 5 s) and a frame every 3 min thereafter until the end (19 × 180 s). Then, ROIs were drawn within the organ boundary in the brain, the pituitary, the nasal mucosa, the parotid gland, the submandibular gland, the thyroid, the ascending aorta artery, the liver, the spleen, the pancreas, the kidney, the adrenal gland, the prostate, and the bone, to obtain TAC data of the tissues. According to our experience in previous studies [19], a reversible 2TCM was used for model fitting, as shown in Fig. 4.18. ^{68}Ga-DOTA-TATE is characterized as a ligand–receptor kinetic tracer; therefore, the meanings of the basic fitting constant rates are different to those of ^{18}F-FDG. Namely, K_1 is associated with the rate of receptor binding, k_2 with the rate of displacement from the receptor, k_3 with the rate of cellular internalization, and k_4 with the rate of externalization. Finally, model fitting to the tissue TAC data was performed, taking the TAC data from ascending aorta artery as the input function. The results for the kinetic metrics are summarized in Table 4.3.

As given in Table 4.3, the rate constants varied dramatically among different organs. Like ^{18}F-FDG, the k_2 constants of ^{68}Ga-DOTA-TATE were much larger than the K_1 constants in most of the organs, potentially indicating a major role of ^{68}Ga-DOTA-TATE clearance within the 60-min time course of dynamic imaging. The exceptional organs were the liver, the spleen, the adrenal gland, the kidney, and the prostate, in which k_2 was relatively smaller than K_1, indicating that the uptake of ^{68}Ga-DOTA-TATE in these organs might remain stable for a long time. Cluster analyses through iterative partitioning with the maxi-

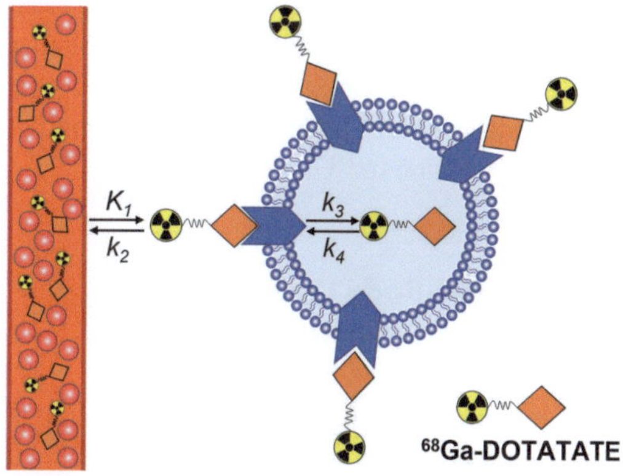

Fig. 4.18 Schematic diagram of the reversible two-tissue compartment for modeling the kinetics of ^{68}Ga-DOTA-TATE. (This figure was adapted from a published open-access article [18])

Table 4.3 Summary statistics of the kinetic metrics of ^{68}Ga-DOTA-TATE in normal organs

Organs	K_1 (mL/min/cm^3)	k_2 (min^{-1})	k_3 (min^{-1})	vB
Nasal mucosa	0.0572 ± 0.0361	0.1025 ± 0.1209	0.0771 ± 0.0747	0.0009 ± 0.0017
Brain	0.2102 ± 0.071	5.4444 ± 2.1166	0.0718 ± 0.0289	0.0021 ± 0.0055
Pituitary	0.1866 ± 0.0425	0.3077 ± 0.8121	1.5915 ± 2.295	0.0195 ± 0.0304
Parotid gland	0.186 ± 0.1476	0.9824 ± 1.7906	0.2817 ± 0.3589	0.0068 ± 0.0069
Submandibular gland	0.2996 ± 0.1646	0.7484 ± 0.5908	0.2091 ± 0.166	0.0233 ± 0.03
Thyroid	0.6024 ± 0.3092	1.5922 ± 1.0735	0.2263 ± 0.1471	0.0152 ± 0.0255
Liver	0.2688 ± 0.0888	0.0926 ± 0.0879	1.2921 ± 2.9613	0.0039 ± 0.0104
Spleen	0.4864 ± 0.1385	0.0174 ± 0.0282	0.0929 ± 0.116	0.014 ± 0.024
Pancreas	0.7439 ± 0.3157	1.9608 ± 0.951	0.246 ± 0.1184	0.0355 ± 0.0442
Kidney	1.1767 ± 0.255	0.3823 ± 0.3048	0.1376 ± 0.1467	0.0076 ± 0.0099
Adrenal gland	0.3657 ± 0.0835	0.1085 ± 0.2728	3.3792 ± 3.0917	0.0862 ± 0.0569
Prostate	0.139 ± 0.0312	0.0594 ± 0.0696	1.5535 ± 3.362	0.0076 ± 0.0171
Bone	0.1532 ± 0.0621	0.5601 ± 0.2665	0.1517 ± 0.0441	0.0089 ± 0.0077

This table was adapted from a published open-access article [18]

mum likelihood criteria were performed to identify organs with similar kinetic characteristics; the results are given in Fig. 4.19.

As given in Fig. 4.19, an optimum of three groups of organs was obtained, according to the kinetic features of ^{68}Ga-DOTA-TATE. The first group had the lowest K_1 and k_3, and the highest k_2, representing low binding and internalization, but high displacement of ^{68}Ga-DOTA-TATE, and consisted of the cerebrum. The second group is consisted of the pituitary gland, the liver, the adrenal gland, and the prostate, which had similar K_1 values to those of the organ in the first group, but with the lowest k_2 and the highest k_3, indicating low displacement and high internalization of ^{68}Ga-DOTA-TATE. The third group had the highest K_1 but a relatively lower k_2 and k_3, including the nasal mucosa, the parotid gland, the submandibular gland, the thyroid, the spleen, the pancreas, the kidney, and the bone, indicating high binding but low internalization of ^{68}Ga-DOTA-TATE.

4.3.3 Total-Body Dynamic PET Imaging in Investigating the Kinetic Distribution Features of ^{68}Ga-PSMA-11 in Normal Organs

The prostate-specific membrane antigen (PSMA) is a type II transmembrane protein that acts as a glutamate carboxypeptidase enzyme. Taking PSMA as target, nuclear medicine imaging has played important role in the diagnosis of prostate cancer and its metastasis, as well as therapeutic strategy decisions for patients. ^{68}Ga-PSMA-11 is a commonly used tracer in the imaging of prostate cancer [20, 21]. However, the physiological uptake of ^{68}Ga-PSMA-11 can be visualized in many organs, such as the prostate, the kidney, the salivary gland, the liver, the spleen, the gastrointestinal tract, the thyroid, and the synovium of the knee. Thus, recognition of the kinetic distribution features of ^{68}Ga-PSMA-11 in normal organs is an important foundation for interpreting ^{68}Ga-PSMA-11 PET images.

Recently, the authors retrospectively enrolled ten patients who had received total-body ^{68}Ga-PSMA-11 dynamic PET imaging, but with non ^{68}Ga-PSMA-11 avid lesions identified on PET images, and no prostate cancerous lesions was identified upon prostate biopsy or in the follow up. All patients underwent 60-min total-body dynamic PET imaging using the long-AFOV uEXPLORER scanner. The dynamic PET data were reconstructed and divided into 55 frames: a frame every 5 s for the initial 3 min (36 × 5 s) and a frame every 3 min thereafter until the end (19 × 180 s). Then, ROIs were drawn within the organ boundary in the parotid gland, the sublingual gland, the submandibular gland, the thyroid, the lung, the descending aorta artery, the myocardium of left ventricle, the liver, the pancreas, the spleen, the kidney, the prostate, the muscle, and the bone, to obtain the TAC data of the tissues. A reversible 2TCM was used for model fitting, in which the meanings of the

Groups	Organs	K_1 (mL/min/cm^3)	k_2 (min^{-1})	k_3 (min^{-1})
1	Brain	0.2102	5.4444	0.0718
2	Pituitary Liver Adrenal gland Prostate	0.2400 ± 0.0861	0.1421 ± 0.0973	1.9541 ± 0.8308
3	Nasal mucosa Parotid gland Submandibular gland Thyroid Spleen Pancreas Kidney Bone	0.4632 ± 0.3486	0.7933 ± 0.6463	0.1778 ± 0.0693

Fig. 4.19 Mean rate constants of organs with similar kinetic features of ^{68}Ga-DOTA-TATE as determined by cluster analysis. (This figure was adapted from a published open-access article [18])

constant rates were similar to those of ^{68}Ga-DOTA-TATE. Finally, model fitting to tissue TAC data was performed, taking the TAC data from descending aorta artery as the input function. The results for the kinetic metrics are summarized in Table 4.4.

As given in Table 4.4, the rate constants varied widely from organ to organ. In all of the organs studied, the k_2 constant was much larger than the K_1 constant, which might indicate that the tissue mainly washed out ^{68}Ga-PSMA-11 during the time course of the dynamic imaging. The liver is particularly distinctive with k_2 (0.401 ± 0.224 min^{-1}) being relatively close to K_1 [0.378 ± 0.124 mL(min cm^3)], which might indicate that the metabolism of ^{68}Ga-PSMA-11 in the normal liver maintains a relatively stable state for a long time. Cluster analyses through iterative partitioning with the maximum likelihood criteria were performed to identify organs with similar kinetic characteristics; the results are given in Fig. 4.20.

As given in Fig. 4.20, an optimum of four groups of organs was obtained according to the kinetic features of ^{68}Ga-PSMA-11. The first group had the largest K_1, k_2, and the smallest k_3, which consisted of the thyroid and the pancreas, representing tissues with the highest vascular density and permeability, and a low expression level of PSMA. The second group consisted of the parotid and the sublingual gland, which showed the largest k_3, a k_2 similar to those of the organs in group 1; however, the K_1 was much smaller. These might indicate a low vascular density, high permeability, and high PSMA expression in these organs. This finding is consistent with the high physiological uptake in the salivary glands. The third group included the lung, the liver, the lumbar spine, the psoas major, and the

Table 4.4 Summary statistics of the kinetic metrics of ^{68}Ga-PSMA-11 in normal organs

Organs	K_1 (mL/min/cm^3)	k_2 (min^{-1})	k_3 (min^{-1})	Ki (mL/cm^3/min)
Thyroid	1.423 ± 0.987	4.337 ± 2.580	0.138 ± 0.072	0.041 ± 0.024
Parotid gland	0.331 ± 0.142	3.512 ± 3.383	3.586 ± 3.337	0.160 ± 0.068
Sublingual gland	0.374 ± 0.216	3.718 ± 2.730	2.409 ± 2.383	0.109 ± 0.028
Submandibular gland	0.604 ± 0.377	3.155 ± 3.145	0.939 ± 0.797	0.165 ± 0.073
Myocardium	0.559 ± 0.399	3.298 ± 2.885	0.892 ± 2.501	0.043 ± 0.078
Lung	0.025 ± 0.053	1.106 ± 2.572	1.423 ± 2.624	0.004 ± 0.003
Spleen	1.391 ± 0.360	2.158 ± 0.862	0.395 ± 0.190	0.214 ± 0.073
Kidney	1.454 ± 0.549	3.180 ± 2.192	1.638 ± 0.840	0.502 ± 0.106
Pancreas	1.049 ± 0.470	3.478 ± 1.447	0.177 ± 0.097	0.049 ± 0.024
Liver	0.378 ± 0.124	0.401 ± 0.224	0.769 ± 1.964	0.117 ± 0.059
Bone	0.213 ± 0.067	0.936 ± 0.316	0.124 ± 0.193	0.017 ± 0.015
Muscle	0.097 ± 0.042	1.152 ± 0.933	0.224 ± 0.417	0.012 ± 0.014
Prostate	0.185 ± 0.046	0.417 ± 0.265	0.168 ± 0.154	0.047 ± 0.012

Groups	Organs	K_1 (mL/min/cm^3)	k_2 (min^{-1})	k_3 (min^{-1})
1	Thyroid Pancreas	1.24	3.91	0.16
2	Parotid gland Sublingual gland	0.35	3.61	3.00
3	Lung Liver Bone Muscle Prostate	0.18	0.80	0.54
4	Submandibular gland Myocardium Spleen Kidney	1.00	2.95	0.97

Fig. 4.20 Mean rate constants of organs with similar kinetic features of ^{68}Ga-PSMA-11 as determined by a cluster analysis

prostate, which had the lowest K_1 and k_2, and a relatively small k_3, indicating low vascular density and permeability, and low PSMA expression in these tissues. The last group, including the submandibular gland, the myocardium, the spleen, and the kidney, which had a K_1 and k_2 similar to those in the organs of the first group, but a larger k_3, which indicated relatively high expression of PSMA and a quicker tissue clearance in these organs.

4.4 Overview and Future Prospects of Tracer Distribution Studies Using Total-Body PET/CT

The application of PET/CT with a long axial FOV has facilitated studies related to PET dynamic imaging; however, they are still in the exploration stage. There are certain problems that remain to be solved, from the dynamic imaging techniques, post-imaging reconstruction, and analysis of dynamic data, to its widespread application in clinics. In addition, the long acquisition time of dynamic imaging, the time-consuming post imaging reconstruction, the complex analysis of dynamic imaging data, and the connection between dynamic PET imaging and pharmacological analysis in clinical pharmacology are also critical difficulties that hinder the promotion and application of dynamic imaging in clinical practice. Herein, we summarize and share our experiences using the total-body PET/CT to explore dynamic imaging studies in our institution.

4.4.1 Caution Regarding Tracer Distribution Studies Using Total-Body PET/CT

4.4.1.1 Plasma Input Curve Conversion

For a radioactive tracer whose transcellular transport can be observed on blood cells (including the red and white blood cells), such as ^{18}F-FDG, its distribution is initially restricted in the plasma immediately after injection, because of the block of the cell membrane. Then, the tracer is gradually distributed to the blood cells via transmembrane transport. After a short time of circulation, the distribution of the tracer will finally achieve equilibrium between the plasma and the blood cells. As mentioned before, only the tracer in a free state in the plasma can be extracted by tissues, but not those trapped in blood cells. Therefore, the measured time-to-activity curve by drawing ROI in large artery of body represents only the time-to-activity curve of the whole blood, namely $C_B(t)$. To obtain the accurate time-to-activity curve of plasma, i.e., $C_p(t)$, for use as the input function, rational correction should be performed to $C_B(t)$. The basic equation to calculate the kinetic constant rates in PET kinetic modeling is expressed as follows:

$$C_{\mathrm{PET}}(t) = vB \times C_B(t) + \left[K_1(1-vB) + vB(k_2+k_3+k_4)\right]\int_0^t C_P(\tau)\,\mathrm{d}\tau$$
$$+\left[vB(k_2 \times k_4) - K_1(k_3+k_4)(1-vB)\right]\int_0^t\int_0^\tau C_P(s)\,\mathrm{d}s\mathrm{d}\tau - (k_2+k_3+k_4)$$
$$\int_0^t C_{\mathrm{PET}}(\tau)\,\mathrm{d}\tau - (k_2 \times k_4)\int_0^t\int_0^\tau C_{\mathrm{PET}}(s)\,\mathrm{d}s\mathrm{d}\tau$$

For this equation, it can be seen that both $C_B(t)$ and $C_p(t)$ are necessary to calculate the kinetic constant rates of K_1–k_4; from this aspect, it is necessary to separate $C_p(t)$ from $C_B(t)$. Taking ^{18}F-FDG as an example, the authors introduced a simple but rational method for converting $C_B(t)$ to $C_p(t)$, which has been proposed in previous studies [22], as follows:

$$C_p(t) = \frac{1-H\left(1-\mathrm{e}^{-at}\right)}{(1-H)}C_B(t)$$

where H denotes the hematocrit, which is recommended to be tested on the same day as PET imaging. If the measured value of H cannot be contained, a mean value of 45% for men and 42.5% for women can be used as an approximation, according to its reference range (40–50% in men, and 37–48% in women) in our country. "a" denotes the constant equilibrium rate, which is about 0.2346 min^{-1} for ^{18}F-FDG [22]. The dynamic change between $C_B(t)$ and $C_p(t)$ is illustrated in Fig. 4.21.

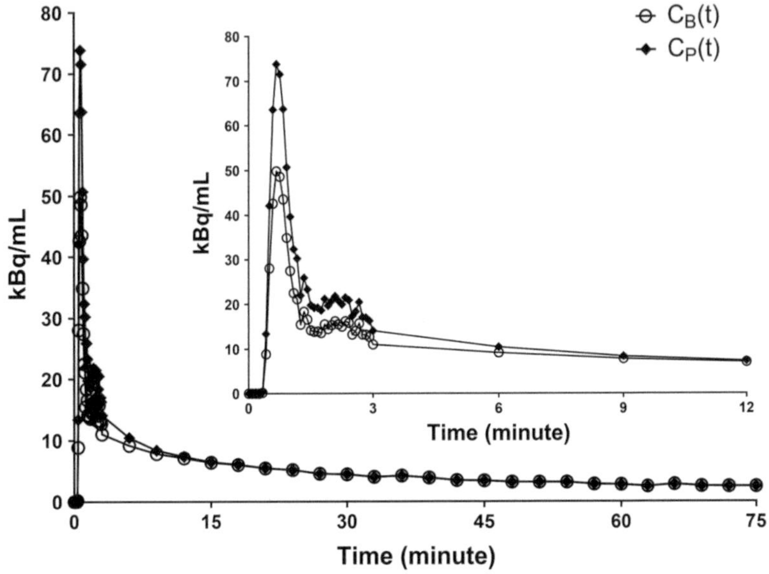

Fig. 4.21 Time course of radioactivity in whole blood [$C_B(t)$] and in corrected plasma [$C_P(t)$] in a typical case. The inserted image illustrates the curves for the first 12 min

4.4.1.2 Time Delay Correction

When dynamic imaging is performed on a traditional PET/CT scanner, the interval between the time when the tracer arrives at the aorta and the time when it arrives in tissue in the field of view can be neglected, because of the limited imaging area. In addition, this tiny time discrepancy can be distinguished by a traditional PET/CT scanner, because of its limited temporal resolution. With the advent of long-AFOV PET/CT scanners, the temporal and spatial resolutions of PET imaging have been significantly improved, and thus tiny discrepancy in time can be captured. Furthermore, dynamic PET imaging is gradually changing from a regional pattern to a simultaneous total-body pattern; therefore, the interval between the time when IDIF begins and the time when tracer arrives in a remote tissue can no longer be neglected. It has been reported that time delay correction could result in significant changes to kinetic metrics, and this phenomenon is more obvious in tissue with a full blood supply. When time delay correction was performed, the vB and K_1 in some organs could increase by up to 69.4% and 4.8%, respectively [23, 24], compared with those calculated without time delay correction. Therefore, time delay correction is recommended when conducting total-body PET kinetic modeling. The exact method and content can be found in the related literature [23, 24].

4.4.1.3 Partial Volume Effect Correction

In brief, the partial volume effect (PVE) occurs when radioactive counts from a source or focus “spill out” into a region that is volumetrically larger in the reconstructed image than its physical size. Although the spatial resolution of long-AFOV PET/CT scanner has significantly improved compared with the traditional PET/CT scanner, it is still significantly lower than that of the traditional imaging modalities, such as CT and MRI. Therefore, the impact of PVE on PET imaging cannot be neglected, which is much more obvious in small lesions. In dynamic imaging, this phenomenon might even be worse, because the counts in each frame of reconstructed PET images are always significantly smaller than those of static PET imaging. The significance of PVE is associated with many factors, including lesion size, shape, circumferent background tracer uptake, and the spatial resolution of the PET scanner [25]. Generally, if the diameter of the lesion is two-fold or more than the spatial resolution of the PET scanner, expressed as full width at half maximum (FWHM) when the point spread function (PSF) is applied, then the PVE can be neglected. As the PSF FWHM of the uEXPLORER system is approximately 3 mm, it is recommended to perform PVE correction for lesions that with diameter less than 6 mm. There are few established methods for PVE correction for lesions in total-body PET imaging. Herein, the authors introduce a simple and widely used method of PVE correction that was established based on data from traditional PET imaging [26]. The equation is expressed as follows:

$$\text{PVE corrected activity} = \frac{\text{Measured activity} - \text{background activity}}{\text{RC}} + \text{background activity}$$

where RC is the recovery coefficient, which is associated with the size of the lesion and the lesion-to-background ratio of tracer uptake, or briefly, it can be searched for in related literature [26].

4.4.2 Future Prospects and Challenges Facing Tracer Distribution Studies Using Total-Body PET/CT

4.4.2.1 Transformation of Pharmacological Kinetics in Clinical Pharmacology

At present, PET kinetic modeling is only applied to investigate the kinetic features of radiopharmaceuticals used for diagnosis or theragnosis. However, for most of the new drugs that are produced mainly for disease treatment, their pharmacokinetic studies are still mainly based on methods from clinical pharmacology. To investigate the kinetic features of these clinical new drugs using dynamic PET imaging and the corresponding kinetic modeling method would be an important application of total-body PET/CT imaging. However, this long-term goal still faces many challenges: (1) Whether the radio-labeled tracer would recover the kinetic features of the clinical new drug remains to be proven by substantial study evidence. (2) Commonly, the clearance half-life of clinical medication can be several hours, which means that repeated PET imaging should be performed several hours after tracer administration, which is a challenge to the traditional PET/CT scanner, given the relative short physical half-lives of the commonly used nuclides in the clinic. Fortunately, this is not a big problem since the advent of total-body PET/CT scanner, thanks to its significantly improved detection sensitivity. (3) Another challenge lies in how to transform the kinetic parameters from PET kinetic modeling to those calculated using clinical pharmacology methods, or how to establish a set of indices that can be used to inform the clinical use of a drug (e.g., drug dosage and the medication interval) based on the kinetic metrics obtained from kinetic modeling.

4.4.2.2 Short Time Dynamic Imaging

An important factor that hinders the widespread use of dynamic PET imaging is the relative long acquisition time. In most of the previous studies regarding dynamic PET imaging, an acquisition time ≥60 min was used, making it difficult to become a routine imaging protocol, especially in those patients with serious diseases who cannot endure long-term immobilization. However, for most of the radioactive tracers, the time to achieve dynamic steady state after injection is less than 60 min, indicating that dynamic PET imaging is not always need to be performed for 60 min. Making use of the improved sensitivity of long-AFOV PET/CT, short time dynamic imaging is a future direction of PET dynamic imaging. Recently, the authors enrolled 11 healthy volunteers to perform dynamic ^{18}F-FDG PET/CT imaging for 75 min. The dynamic data of each patient was then divided into the first 30-min group, the 45-min group, and the entire 75-min group. The same methods to determine the same parameter configurations of kinetic modeling were applied to these data to calculate the kinetic metrics. Comparable results for the kinetic metrics in normal organs were identified between the 45-min group and 75-min group, which indicated that an acquisition time of 45 min is sufficient for dynamic imaging to investigate the kinetic metrics of ^{18}F-FDG in normal tissues [6]. For tumors, especially those with high tracer uptake, tracer distribution would achieve a dynamic steady state even faster, indicating that the required acquisition time might be even shorter. This phenomenon also applies to some tracers that feature fast kinetics, such as the fibroblast activation protein inhibitor (FAPI), which has demonstrated great potential for widespread use in clinics. However, these observations require further clinical validation.

4.4.2.3 Capture of Early Kinetic Features

The TOF temporal resolution of the uEXPLORER scanner is about 430 ps. Therefore, if making use of the Kernel maximum expectation algorithm, PET imaging can capture the sub-second pathophysiological changes of organic bodies [27]. This technical improvement might facilitate the application of dynamic PET imaging in the future in the following areas: (1) To assess blood flow perfusion in tissues or organs through studying the kinetic features of some radionuclides with fast metabolism, such as ^{82}Rb, ^{13}N, and ^{15}O; (2) to capture the early dynamic changes of a tracer to investigate the first-pass information of the tracer using 1TCM kinetic modeling, which can be used to improve diagnosis efficiency, in combination with static imaging performed at a relatively later time [28]; (3) to capture and freeze the process of physiological motion (e.g., the heartbeat, respiratory movement, and intestinal peristalsis) to investigate the biomechanical-kinetic features of organs; (4) to visualize the simultaneous dynamic molecular changes of organs over the entire body to reveal inter-organ correlations in organic bodies, such as the brain-heart axis and the brain-gut axis [29].

4.4.2.4 Multiple Parametric Imaging

With the advance of medical techniques and the improved requirements for precision medicine, single-mode imaging is no longer able to fulfill the clinical requirement for "early detection, early diagnosis and early treatment" of diseases. Technological breakthroughs have been achieved in obtaining static SUV images accompanied by a set of kinetic parametric images through single dynamic PET imaging by using the long-AFOV PET/CT scanner. Thus, in the near future, the working pattern of nuclear physicians would change from reading a single set of static SUV images to comparing and analyzing patterns of multiple parametric images in addition to static SUV images. These patterns will be helpful to obtaining multi-dimensional metabolic information of the tracer from multiple angles and multiple levels, which will promote a deeper recognition of pathophysiological changes of diseases and precision medicine, similar to the patterns of multiple-sequence, multiple-parameter magnetic resonance imaging. Therefore, how to read the parametric images accurately, to recognize their interrelationships, to understand the connections between underlying mechanisms and pathophysiological changes of diseases, and to handle the daily working burden of reading such a huge number of images represent the challenges facing nuclear medicine physicians in the future.

In conclusion, with the improvement of equipment and techniques of long-AFOV PET/CT scanners, the detection sensitivity, temporal resolution, and spatial resolution of PET imaging has been significantly improved, which has greatly facilitated the promotion and widespread clinical application of dynamic PET imaging. The pattern of dynamic PET imaging has also changed from the traditional single-bed imaging or multiple-bed multiple-pass imaging to simultaneous total-body dynamic imaging. Therefore, for any new radioactive tracer, the total-body dynamic PET imaging using the long-AFOV PET/CT scanner can be carried out to investigate its pharmacological characteristics before putting to clinical use, which might serve as a reference for detailed study of the tracer and deeper interpretation of the images. Moreover, the long-AFOV PET/CT scanner has opened new fields of application and study for dynamic PET imaging, such as investigating the kinetic features of clinical new drugs, to perform dynamic PET imaging with reduced acquisition time, to capture early pharmacokinetic features of the tracer, and to conduct multiple parametric PET imaging. However, the promotion and widespread application of dynamic PET imaging is still facing various challenges, for instance, how to transform and connect PET kinetic modeling methods and the corresponding kinetic metrics to the pharmacokinetic method in clinical pharmacology and the corresponding kinetic parameters; how to extract valuable features from the abundant information from dynamic PET imaging and the corresponding pharmacokinetic analysis for an enhanced contribution to clinical practice; and how to handle the huge working burden facing nuclear physicians in the future regarding the interpretation of multiple parametric images obtained from dynamic PET imaging.

References

1. Dunnwald LK, Doot RK, Specht JM, Gralow JR, Ellis GK, Livingston RB, et al. PET tumor metabolism in locally advanced breast cancer patients undergoing neoadjuvant chemotherapy: value of static versus kinetic measures of fluorodeoxyglucose uptake. Clin Cancer Res. 2011;17(8):2400–9.
2. Doot RK, Kurland BF, Kinahan PE, Mankoff DA. Design considerations for using PET as a response measure in single site and multicenter clinical trials. Acad Radiol. 2012;19(2):184–90.
3. Badawi RD, Shi H, Hu P, Chen S, Xu T, Price PM, et al. First human imaging studies with the EXPLORER total-body PET scanner. J Nucl Med. 2019;60(3):299–303.
4. Alberts I, Hunermund JN, Prenosil G, Mingels C, Bohn KP, Viscione M, et al. Clinical performance of long axial field of view PET/CT: a head-to-head intra-individual comparison of the Biograph Vision Quadra with the Biograph Vision PET/CT. Eur J Nucl Med Mol Imaging. 2021;48(8):2395–404.
5. Velikyan I, Sundin A, Sorensen J, Lubberink M, Sandstrom M, Garske-Roman U, et al. Quantitative and qualitative intrapatient comparison of ^{68}Ga-DOTATOC and ^{68}Ga-DOTATATE: net uptake rate for accurate quantification. J Nucl Med. 2014;55(2):204–10.
6. Liu G, Yu H, Shi D, Hu P, Hu Y, Tan H, et al. Short-time total-body dynamic PET imaging performance in quantifying the kinetic metrics of ^{18}F-FDG in healthy volunteers. Eur J Nucl Med Mol Imaging. 2022;49(8):2493–503.
7. Torizuka T, Nobezawa S, Momiki S, Kasamatsu N, Kanno T, Yoshikawa E, et al. Short dynamic FDG-PET imaging protocol for patients with lung cancer. Eur J Nucl Med. 2000;27(10):1538–42.
8. Foster B, Bagci U, Mansoor A, Xu Z, Mollura DJ. A review on segmentation of positron emission tomography images. Comput Biol Med. 2014;50:76–96.
9. Dimitrakopoulou-Strauss A, Strauss LG, Heichel T, Wu H, Burger C, Bernd L, et al. The role of quantitative ^{18}F-FDG PET studies for the differentiation of malignant and benign bone lesions. J Nucl Med. 2002;43(4):510–8.
10. Dimitrakopoulou-Strauss A, Strauss LG, Schwarzbach M, Burger C, Heichel T, Willeke F, et al. Dynamic PET ^{18}F-FDG studies in patients with primary and recurrent soft-tissue sarcomas: impact on diagnosis and correlation with grading. J Nucl Med. 2001;42(5):713–20.
11. Strauss LG, Dimitrakopoulou-Strauss A, Koczan D, Bernd L, Haberkorn U, Ewerbeck V, et al. ^{18}F-FDG kinetics and gene expression in giant cell tumors. J Nucl Med. 2004,45(9):1528–35.
12. Morita K, Katoh C, Yoshinaga K, Noriyasu K, Mabuchi M, Tsukamoto T, et al. Quantitative analysis of myocardial glucose utilization in patients with left ventricular dysfunction by means of ^{18}F-FDG dynamic positron tomography and three-compartment analysis. Eur J Nucl Med Mol Imaging. 2005;32(7):806–12.
13. Yokoyama I, Inoue Y, Moritan T, Ohtomo K, Nagai R. Measurement of skeletal muscle glucose utilization by dynamic ^{18}F-FDG PET without arterial blood sampling. Nucl Med Commun. 2005;26(1):31–7.
14. Tilsley DW, Harte RJ, Jones T, Brady F, Luthra SK, Brown G, et al. New techniques in the pharmacokinetic analysis of cancer drugs. IV. Positron emission tomography. Cancer Surv. 1993;17:425–42.
15. Fujimura Y, Kimura Y, Simeon FG, Dickstein LP, Pike VW, Innis RB, et al. Biodistribution and radiation dosimetry in humans of a new PET ligand, ^{18}F-PBR06, to image translocator protein (18 kDa). J Nucl Med. 2010;51(1):145–9.
16. Rahmim A, Lodge MA, Karakatsanis NA, Panin VY, Zhou Y, McMillan A, et al. Dynamic whole-body PET imaging: principles, potentials and applications. Eur J Nucl Med Mol Imaging. 2019;46(2):501–18.
17. Liu G, Xu H, Hu P, Tan H, Zhang Y, Yu H, et al. Kinetic metrics of ^{18}F-FDG in normal human organs identified by systematic dynamic total-body positron emission tomography. Eur J Nucl Med Mol Imaging. 2021;48(8):2363–72.
18. Yin H, Liu G, Hu Y, Xiao J, Mao W, Lv J, et al. Dynamic total-body PET/CT imaging reveals kinetic distribution of ^{68}Ga-DOTATATE in normal organs. Contrast Media Mol Imaging. 2023;2023:4722499.
19. Henze M, Dimitrakopoulou-Strauss A, Milker-Zabel S, Schuhmacher J, Strauss LG, Doll J, et al. Characterization of ^{68}Ga-DOTA-D-Phe1-Tyr3--octreotide kinetics in patients with meningiomas. J Nucl Med. 2005;46(5):763–9.
20. Fendler WP, Eiber M, Beheshti M, Bomanji J, Ceci F, Cho S, et al. ^{68}Ga-PSMA PET/CT: joint EANM and SNMMI procedure guideline for prostate cancer imaging: version 1.0. Eur J Nucl Med Mol Imaging. 2017;44(6):1014–24.
21. Backhaus P, Noto B, Avramovic N, Grubert LS, Huss S, Bogemann M, et al. Targeting PSMA by radioligands in non-prostate disease-current status and future perspectives. Eur J Nucl Med Mol Imaging. 2018;45(5):860–77.

22. Wahl LM, Asselin MC, Nahmias C. Regions of interest in the venous sinuses as input functions for quantitative PET. J Nucl Med. 1999;40(10):1666–75.
23. Li EJ, Spencer BA, Schmall JP, Abdelhafez Y, Badawi RD, Wang G, et al. Efficient delay correction for total-body PET kinetic modeling using pulse timing methods. J Nucl Med. 2022;63(8):1266–73.
24. Wang G, Nardo L, Parikh M, Abdelhafez YG, Li E, Spencer BA, et al. Total-body PET multiparametric imaging of cancer using a voxel-wise strategy of compartmental modeling. J Nucl Med. 2022;63(8):1274–81.
25. Soret M, Bacharach SL, Buvat I. Partial-volume effect in PET tumor imaging. J Nucl Med. 2007;48(6):932–45.
26. Srinivas SM, Dhurairaj T, Basu S, Bural G, Surti S, Alavi A. A recovery coefficient method for partial volume correction of PET images. Ann Nucl Med. 2009;23(4):341–8.
27. Zhang X, Cherry SR, Xie Z, Shi H, Badawi RD, Qi J. Subsecond total-body imaging using ultrasensitive positron emission tomography. Proc Natl Acad Sci U S A. 2020;117(5):2265–7.
28. Feng T, Zhao Y, Shi H, Li H, Zhang X, Wang G, et al. Total-body quantitative parametric imaging of early kinetics of ^{18}F-FDG. J Nucl Med. 2021;62(5):738–44.
29. Mayer EA. Gut feelings: the emerging biology of gut-brain communication. Nat Rev Neurosci. 2011;12(8):453–66.

Interpretation and Application of Total-Body PET/CT Dynamic Acquisition Information

5

Yibo He, Yiqiu Zhang, Danjie Cai, Jing Lv, Haojun Yu, and Hongcheng Shi

The total-body positron emission tomography–computed tomography (TB PET/CT) technique is capable of completing total-body dynamic imaging because of its ultra-long axial field of view, high sensitivity, and high temporal resolution. Real-time dynamic image analysis based on total-body imaging not only enables visualization of pharmacokinetics, but also allows for parametric imaging, and the evaluation of blood supply, distribution processes, and states of target tissues or organs using time-activity curves (TACs) of target tissues or organs. Valuable biological information can be obtained through these methods.

5.1 Total-Body PET/CT Parametric Imaging and Its Application

PET is a non-invasive quantitative imaging tool that dynamically monitors the spatial and temporal distribution of radiotracers in the human body, providing insights into the physiology of tissues. Compared with static PET imaging, the use of tracer kinetic modeling to simulate the spatial and temporal distribution of radiotracers in the body allows the quantification of physiologically meaningful parameters, resulting in the generation of parametric images of radiotracer kinetics. These parametric images display the dynamic parameter values corresponding to each image voxel, effectively reflecting the uptake of tracers by different tissues [1].

The pharmacokinetic model is based on a quantitative mathematical model that simulates a series of biochemical reactions following the injection of a radiotracer into the body. By combining PET image data with the collected physiological data, the kinetic parameters of tissues can be estimated. This process is divided into three steps: the establishment of a mathematical model, the derivation of input and output functions, and parameter estimation.

The compartmental model is a classic pharmacokinetic model that is commonly used to describe the distribution of radiotracers in the body. This model refers to a state in which the radiotracer may exist, rather than a fixed anatomical structure. Therefore, a compartment can be composed of different biological tissues, and the same biological tissue may also contain multiple compartments, with the radiotracer entering and leaving at a specific rate. This model is relatively simple and can effectively quantify the physiological parameters of specific regions from PET data. The three basic elements of the compartmental model are the input function, output function, and kinetic parameters [2]. The input function represents the process by which the concentration of radiotracers in the plasma changes over time. Arterial blood sampling is the "gold

Y. He · Y. Zhang · D. Cai · J. Lv · H. Yu · H. Shi (✉)
Department of Nuclear Medicine, Zhongshan Hospital, Fudan University, Shanghai, China
e-mail: shi.hongcheng@zs-hospital.sh.cn

© Shanghai Scientific and Technical Publishers 2024
H. Shi et al. (eds.), *Total-Body PET/CT*, https://doi.org/10.1007/978-981-97-5065-8_5

standard" to obtain the input function. However, to avoid the risks associated with invasive operations, researchers have proposed an image-derived input function (IDIF) method, which involves outlining regions of interest (ROIs) in blood pools, such as the left ventricle, left atrium, and aorta, to obtain the input function for pharmacokinetic modeling and parameter estimation [3, 4]. The output function represents the TAC of the tissue, which can be obtained by directly outlining the target tissue on the PET dynamic scan image. Based on the determined input function, output function, and kinetic model, different tissue-specific kinetic parameters can be obtained through data fitting.

Studies have demonstrated that the Patlak analysis, a graphical analysis method based on the linearization of irreversible compartmental models, could be considered the "gold standard" of kinetic models [5, 6]. This method calculates the net influx rate constant (K_i) of the tracer based on the target tissue TAC, pharmacokinetic model, and plasma glucose level, and it is relatively easy to obtain K_i parametric images [7]. It has been shown that K_i parametric images can improve lesion detection by inhibiting the physiological distribution of ^{18}F-fluorodeoxyglucose (FDG) in the blood pool, leading to higher contrast in the abnormal uptake areas of the lesion [8, 9]. Consequently, when the ^{18}F-FDG uptake in tumors is low or the lesion is located in tissues or organs with high physiological uptake (such as the liver), lesion detection using K_i parametric images is superior to static PET images (Fig. 5.1). However, for tissues or organs with low physiological uptake of the radiotracers and lesions with much higher uptake of the radiotracers than the surrounding background tissue, K_i parametric imaging does not show significant advantages in lesion detection. Nevertheless, K_i parametric images have a higher tumor-to-background ratio (TBR), which improves diagnostic accuracy (Fig. 5.2).

Currently, various PET parameter imaging methods based on both linear graphical models (such as the Patlak model and Logan model) and non-linear kinetic models have been established. These methods include both indirect and direct reconstruction. Indirect reconstruction involves reconstructing PET data frame by frame to obtain the radioactivity distribution images at each time point, followed by fitting a pharmacokinetic

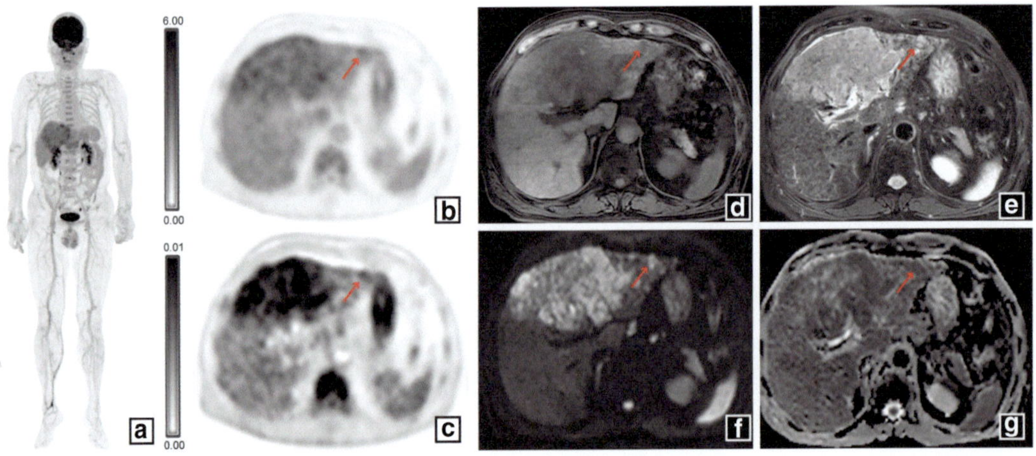

Fig. 5.1 Low-dose parametric image of a patient with malignant liver tumor. A 63-year-old male patient underwent half-dose (1.85 MBq/kg) ^{18}F-FDG TB PET/CT dynamic imaging for 75 min, followed by the reconstruction of 15-min static PET images (**a**, maximum intensity projection (MIP); **b**, transverse) and K_i parametric images (**c**, transverse). The liver lesion located in the left lobe, which was indistinct on the static image, but exhibited abnormal uptake of ^{18}F-FDG on the K_i parametric image (indicated by the arrows). On the same day, the patient underwent an ^{18}F-FDG PET/magnetic resonance (MR) examination, where the lesion was visualized on a T_1 weighted image (T_1WI) (**d**), T_2WI (**e**), diffusion weighted image (DWI) (**f**), and apparent diffusion coefficient (ADC) (**g**) images

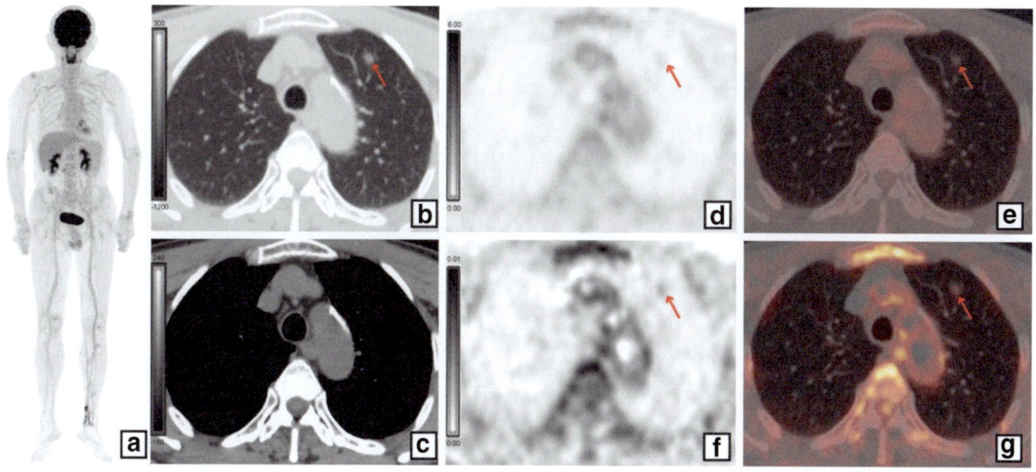

Fig. 5.2 Parametric image of left lung adenocarcinoma. A 70-year-old male patient underwent ultra-low dose (0.37 MBq/kg) ^{18}F-FDG TB PET/CT dynamic imaging for 75 min. Images were reconstructed into a 15-min PET static image (**a**, MIP), CT images of lung window (**b**), and mediastinal window (**c**), PET image (**d**), and PET/CT fusion image (**e**), as well as a K_i parametric PET image (**f**) and its fusion image (**g**). The arrows indicate a lesion located in the left upper lobe of the lung, which exhibited a TBR of 3.1 and 5.7 on the static and K_i PET images, respectively. The postoperative pathology revealed a diagnosis of invasive lung adenocarcinoma with a differentiation grade of II

model to the TAC on each voxel to obtain parametric images. This method is relatively easy to implement and computationally simple. However, the noise distribution in the reconstructed images is difficult to model, resulting in higher noise in the parametric images [10]. In contrast, direct reconstruction combines the tracer kinetic model and PET image reconstruction model into one mathematical problem, allowing it to directly derive parametric images from dynamic PET data, while modeling noise distribution in the reconstructed images. This approach can yield more accurate estimates of pharmacokinetic parameters from dynamic PET sinograms, making it a preferable alternative to indirect reconstruction.

5.2 Application of TAC in the Differential Diagnosis of Liver Tumors

Parametric imaging with PET has been widely used in various fields, such as oncology, cardiology, and neurology [11–13]. Despite its widespread use, parametric imaging still faces numerous challenges. Firstly, dynamic acquisition requires a long scanning time (typically 60 min), which can impede overall clinical efficiency. For patients who have difficulties remaining motionless for a long time, such as children or critically ill patients, long scans can easily result in motion artifacts, thus affecting image quality. Secondly, there is a certain risk associated with obtaining the input function through arterial blood sampling, and non-invasively deriving an accurate input function is also a current research challenge. Furthermore, considering the dual blood supply of the liver, the estimation of kinetic parameters also needs to include tracer inputs from both the hepatic artery and the portal vein. Although liver parametric imaging has increased value compared with static PET images, current kinetic models based on single input functions might result in an overall underestimation of their kinetic parameters.

A retrospective analysis of 109 patients with hepatocellular carcinoma (HCC), intrahepatic cholangiocarcinoma (ICC), and colorectal cancer with liver metastasis (CRLM) was conducted based on dynamic imaging TAC features obtained from 60-min TB PET/CT dynamic imaging. The dynamic scans were divided into two phases: a perfusion phase (first 3 min, 5 s/frame) and a metabolism phase (last 57 min, 3 min/frame). The arterial phase was defined as 15 s after the peak activity of the hepatic artery in the perfusion phase, and rapid progression was defined as TBR >1.5 for the frame in the arterial phase. The metabolic tumor TAC was classified into three types (A, B, and C) (Fig. 5.3). Type A showed a sustained increase, Type B showed a gradual decrease over the first 30 min (approaching the background liver activity) followed by a gradual increase over the next 30 min, and Type C showed a gradual decrease over the whole course. TBR was calculated by dividing the tumor activity by the background liver activity, with TBR_{30} (27–30 min after injection) and TBR_{60} (57–60 min after injection) being calculated for the reconstructed images. $TBR_{30/60}$ was defined as (TBR_{60}-TBR_{30})/TBR_{30}, and Type C images were excluded from the $TBR_{30/60}$ calculations. The results showed that the use of rapid progression as a diagnostic criterion for HCC yielded a sensitivity, specificity, positive predictive value, and negative predictive value of 66.7%, 75.6%, 48.6%, and 86.8%, respectively. Furthermore, the use of the Type B curve as a diagnostic criterion for HCC yielded a specificity and negative predictive value of 82.9% and 82.4%, respectively. The findings of this study indicated that combining TAC with $TBR_{30/60}$ obtained from TB PET/CT dynamic imaging provides additional diagnostic value for liver tumors and is an effective complement to static PET/CT imaging [14].

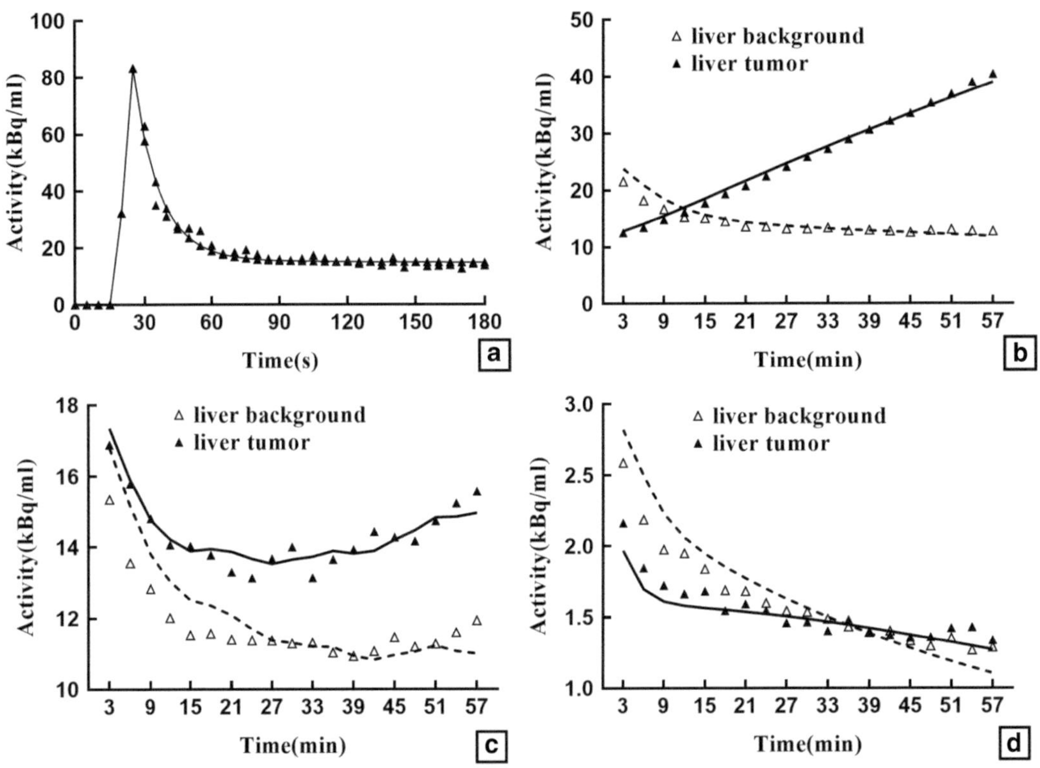

Fig. 5.3 Types of TACs illustrating metabolic tumor phases. (**a**) Normal aorta TAC, showing a sharp single peak. (**b**) Type A curve, with a continuous increase in tumor TAC from 3 to 60 min. (**c**) Type B curve, with a gradual decrease in tumor TAC from 3 to 30 min (similar to the liver background trend), followed by a gradual increase after 30 min. (**d**) Type C curve, with a gradual decrease in tumor TAC over the entire course. (This figure was adapted with permission from a published article (Adili et al. [14]))

5.3 Evaluation of Organ Function Using TB PET/CT Dynamic Imaging

Dynamic imaging with TB PET/CT provides rich information, allowing for the observation of the physiological distribution of radiotracers within different organs and the dynamic evaluation of functional changes in target organs before and after certain interventions.

Prostate Specific Membrane Antigen (PSMA) is a type II transmembrane glycoprotein that is mainly expressed in prostate tissue and is highly expressed in most primary and metastatic prostate cancers. Therefore, integrated diagnosis and treatment targeting PSMA receptors have been developed in clinical practice. ^{68}Ga-PSMA-11 is widely used because of its high uptake in tumor tissue, rapid blood clearance, and low liver background, and is employed not only for diagnosis, but also for predicting the in vivo distribution of therapeutic drugs, such as ^{177}Lu-PSMA.

Our team explored the feasibility of reducing the accumulation of ^{68}Ga-PSMA-11 in salivary glands during TB PET/CT dynamic imaging by orally administering vitamin C, to minimize radiation damage to the salivary glands during the use of therapeutic radiopharmaceuticals [15]. Salivary glands show a high physiological uptake of ^{68}Ga-PSMA-11, which poses a potential risk of causing xerostomia when using radiopharmaceuticals labeled with β or α particles targeting PSMA for the treatment of metastatic prostate cancer.

Between October 2020 and March 2021, 31 patients with prostate cancer underwent low-dose TB PET/CT. All patients received a foot vein injection of ^{68}Ga-PSMA-11 (0.027 mCi/kg) and underwent 60-min total-body dynamic imaging. Among them, 11 patients were randomly assigned to the experimental group and given 400 mg of oral vitamin C during dynamic acquisition at 30 min, while the remaining 20 patients served as the control group and did not receive vitamin C. The raw data were reconstructed into 55 frames of images, with the first 36 frames reconstructed at 5 s per frame and the last 19 frames reconstructed at 180 s per frame. Subsequently, volumes of interest (VOIs) were delineated using automated segmentation software on the reconstructed PET static images, and TACs were obtained for both the bilateral parotid and submandibular glands. The mean standardized uptake value (SUVmean) of the VOIs was recorded on the 60-min (55th frame) PET image, and the trend of the SUVmean from 30 to 60 min was calculated.

Analysis of the 55th frame of the PET static image revealed that the SUVmean values of the bilateral parotid and submandibular glands in the experimental group of patients with prostate cancer were 15.4 ± 3.1, 15.0 ± 2.6, 14.9 ± 4.4, and 15.4 ± 4.2 for the left and right sides, respectively, while in the control group, they were 19.4 ± 3.8, 20.1 ± 3.6, 22.6 ± 5.6, and 22.7 ± 5.9 respectively. Statistical analysis revealed a significant difference in SUVmean between the two groups ($p < 0.001$). The SUVmean of the bilateral parotid and submandibular glands on the left and right sides in the experimental group decreased by 26%, 34%, 52%, and 48%, respectively, compared with those in the control group. The slopes from 30 to 60 min were 0.63 ± 0.13, 0.64 ± 0.14, 0.56 ± 0.25, and 0.62 ± 0.26 for the bilateral parotid and submandibular glands in the experimental group, and 0.84 ± 0.21, 0.84 ± 0.17, 1.01 ± 0.34, and 1.02 ± 0.37 for the control group, respectively. Statistical analysis revealed a significant difference in the trend of changes between the two groups (all $p < 0.05$). These findings suggested that TB PET/CT dynamic imaging can effectively evaluate the dynamic changes in the function of target tissues or organs (Fig. 5.4).

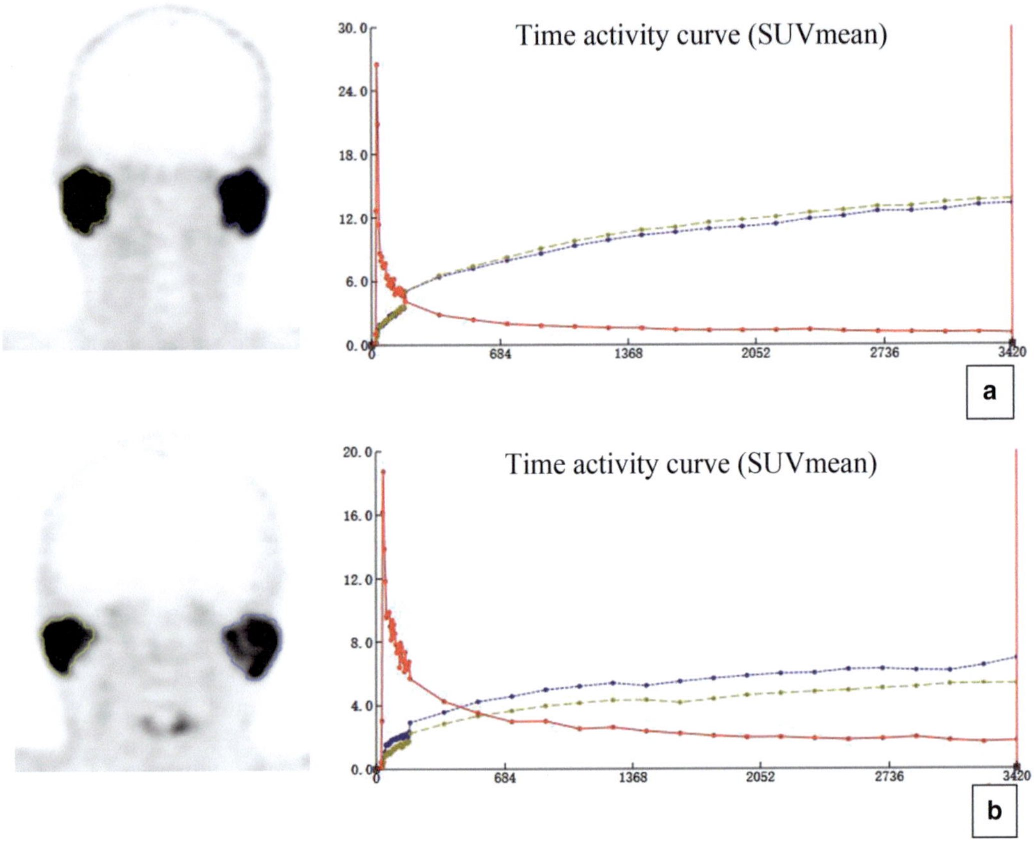

Fig. 5.4 TACs of salivary gland uptake of ^{68}Ga-PSMA-11. Dynamic imaging of ^{68}Ga-PSMA-11 using TB PET/CT. (**a**) TACs of bilateral parotid glands in the control group. (**b**) TACs of bilateral parotid glands in the experimental group with oral administration of vitamin C at 30 min. The slope of TACs between 30 and 60 min in the experimental group with oral administration of vitamin C was significantly lower than that of the group without vitamin C

References

1. Wang G, Qi J. Direct estimation of kinetic parametric images for dynamic PET. Theranostics. 2013;3(10):802–15.
2. Bertoldo A, Peltoniemi P, Oikonen V, et al. Kinetic modeling of [^{18}F] FDG in skeletal muscle by PET: a four-compartment five-rate-constant model. Am J Physiol Endocrinol Metab. 2001;281(3):E524–36.
3. van der Weerdt AP, Klein LJ, Boellaard R, et al. Image-derived input functions for determination of MRGlu in cardiac ^{18}F-FDG PET scans. J Nucl Med. 2001;42(11):1622–9.
4. Sari H, Mingels C, Alberts I, et al. First results on kinetic modelling and parametric imaging of dynamic ^{18}F-FDG datasets from a long axial FOV PET scanner in oncological patients. Eur J Nucl Med Mol Imaging. 2022;49(6):1997–2009.
5. Dimitrakopoulou-Strauss A, Pan L, Sachpekidis C. Parametric imaging with dynamic PET for oncological applications: protocols, interpretation, current applications and limitations for clinical use. Semin Nucl Med. 2022;52(3):312–29.
6. Dias AH, Pedersen MF, Danielsen H, et al. Clinical feasibility and impact of fully automated multiparametric PET imaging using direct Patlak reconstruction: evaluation of 103 dynamic whole-body ^{18}F-FDG PET/CT scans. Eur J Nucl Med Mol Imaging. 2021;48(3):837–50.
7. Yang M, Lin Z, Xu Z, et al. Influx rate constant of ^{18}F-FDG increases in metastatic lymph nodes of non-small cell lung cancer patients. Eur J Nucl Med Mol Imaging. 2020;47(5):1198–208.
8. Fahrni G, Karakatsanis NA, Di Domenicantonio G, et al. Does whole-body Patlak ^{18}F-FDG PET imaging improve lesion detectability in clinical oncology? Eur Radiol. 2019;29(9):4812–21.

9. Zaker N, Kotasidis F, Garibotto V, et al. Assessment of lesion detectability in dynamic whole-body PET imaging using compartmental and Patlak parametric mapping. Clin Nucl Med. 2020;45(5):e221–31.
10. Zhang X, Xie Z, Berg E, et al. Total-body dynamic reconstruction and parametric imaging on the uEXPLORER. J Nucl Med. 2020;61(2):285–91.
11. Baker SL, Lockhart SN, Price JC, et al. Reference tissue-based kinetic evaluation of ^{18}F-AV-1451 for tau imaging. J Nucl Med. 2017;58(2):332–8.
12. Wang T, Wu KY, Miner RC, et al. Reproducible quantification of cardiac sympathetic innervation using graphical modeling of carbon-11-metahydroxyephedrine kinetics with dynamic PET-CT imaging. EJNMMI Res. 2018;8(1):63.
13. Ilan E, Sandström M, Velikyan I, et al. Parametric net influx rate images of ^{68}Ga-DOTATOC and ^{68}Ga-DOTATATE: quantitative accuracy and improved image contrast. J Nucl Med. 2017;58(5):744–9.
14. Adili D, Cai D, Cao Y, et al. Added value of ^{18}F-FDG total-body PET/CT dynamic imaging in the diagnosis of liver malignant tumors. Chin J Nucl Med Mol Imaging. 2022;42(12):724–8.
15. Lv J, Yin H, Yu H, et al. The feasibility of ultralow-activity ^{18}F-FDG dynamic PET imaging in lung adenocarcinoma patients through total-body PET/CT scanner. Ann Nucl Med. 2022;36(10):887–96.

Clinical Application of Low-Dose Total-Body PET/CT Scan

6

Hui Tan, Yibo He, Danjie Cai, and Dilibire Adili

Conventional positron emission tomography–computed tomography (PET/CT) has a 15–30 cm axial field of view and often recommends a minimum image acquisition of 7 MBq/kg/min/bed [1, 2]. This translates to 2 min/bed for image acquisition and a standard dose of approximately 3.7 MBq/kg for ^{18}F-fluorodeoxyglucose (FDG). With a 194-cm extra-long axial field of view, total-body (TB) PET/CT offers significantly increased system sensitivity, allowing for low-dose PET imaging. Half-dose PET imaging involves injecting only 1.85 MBq/kg instead of the recommended dose of 3.7 MBq/kg ^{18}F-FDG, thereby reducing radiopharmaceutical costs, and enabling more patients to undergo imaging with limited ^{18}F-FDG supply. Additionally, administering lower doses of imaging agents can lessen the radiation exposure risks for medical personnel during the procedures and has fewer irradiation effects on patients.

6.1 Feasibility Study of Half-Dose TB PET/CT Imaging

6.1.1 Comparative Study of Half-Dose ^{18}F-FDG TB PET/CT Versus Conventional PET/CT Imaging

To confirm the viability of utilizing half-dose ^{18}F-FDG TB PET/CT imaging in clinical settings, a comparative study was conducted on patients with lung cancer [3]. The study compared patients who underwent half-dose ^{18}F-FDG TB PET/CT imaging with those who received conventional digital PET/CT imaging. In total, 28 patients with confirmed primary lung cancer underwent the half-dose (1.85 MBq/kg) ^{18}F-FDG TB PET/CT (uEXPLORER) before therapy. In the conventional digital PET/CT (uMI780) group, 28 patients with lung cancer who received full-dose (3.70 MBq/kg) ^{18}F-FDG with imaging acquisi-

H. Tan (✉) · Y. He · D. Cai · D. Adili
Department of Nuclear Medicine, Zhongshan Hospital, Fudan University, Shanghai, China
e-mail: tan.hui@zs-hospital.sh.cn

© Shanghai Scientific and Technical Publishers 2024
H. Shi et al. (eds.), *Total-Body PET/CT*, https://doi.org/10.1007/978-981-97-5065-8_6

tion for 2 min/bed were selected from the database. Image quality in PET is influenced by various factors such as instrumentation, imaging and reconstruction parameters, imaging agents, subject preparation, and individual subject characteristics, such blood glucose levels, history of diabetes, and body mass index (BMI). As a result, comparing PET images across different groups requires careful consideration of these factors. For this study, we ensured that the conventional digital PET/CT group and the half-dose ^{18}F-FDG TB PET/CT group were matched in terms of age, sex, BMI, history of diabetes, waiting time after injection, type of lung cancer pathology, and lesion size, to ensure a fair comparison. The conventional digital uMI780 PET/CT has a 30-cm axial field of view and is produced by the same manufacturer as the ultra-long axial field of view TB PET/CT instrument, which can be regarded as a "microscopic version" of TB PET uEXPLORER. Apart from the different axial field of view, they have basically the same hardware configuration.

The TB PET/CT scanner was employed in the 3D list mode to continuously perform PET scans for a duration of 15 min in the half-dose group. PET images were reconstructed using all 15 min of data and were also reconstructed into 4-min and 2-min images, known as G15, G4, and G2, respectively. For comparison purposes, we selected the reconstructed 4-min and 2-min images to compare with conventional digital PET/CT, which involved full-dose ^{18}F-FDG group acquisition at a speed of 2 min/bed. The conventional digital PET/CT scans ranged from the roof of the skull to the middle of the femur, employing time of flight (TOF) and point spread function (PSF) modeling, three iterations and 20 subsets, matrix 192 × 192, slice thickness of 1.443 mm, and the Gaussian filter function 3 mm as the parameters for reconstructing PET images using the ordered subset expectation maximization (OSEM) algorithm.

The quality of the PET images was assessed using both subjective and objective indicators. For the subjective analysis, a 5-point Likert scale was used, with ratings ranging from 1 (poor) to 5 (excellent): 1, inferior image quality; 2, poor image quality; 3, average image quality; 4, good image quality; and 5, excellent image quality. Image quality scores of 3 or higher were deemed acceptable for clinical diagnostic purposes. The PET images were evaluated independently by two experienced nuclear radiologists who had been practicing nuclear medicine for at least 5 years. Objective image quality was evaluated using semi-quantitative indicators such as maximum standard uptake value (SUV_{max}), mean standard uptake value (SUV_{mean}), and signal-to-noise ratio (SNR) of the liver and mediastinal blood pool. To calculate the liver's background uptake value, a manually drawn region of interest (ROI) with a diameter of 20 mm was outlined at the portal vein bifurcation in the liver's right lobe, avoiding visible lesions and large intrahepatic vessels. To assess the background uptake values of the mediastinal blood pool, an ROI of similar size or appropriately reduced in size was selected on the ascending aorta at the bronchial bifurcation while avoiding the vessel wall. The SNR was calculated as the SUV_{mean} divided by its standard deviation (SD). G15 was used as the reference standard for G2 and G4 detection of lesions.

Based on the findings of the PET image subjective score, the mean and SD of the image quality scores were calculated for G2, G4, and G15 in the half-dose group. The scores for G2, G4, and G15 were 4.3 ± 0.7, 4.9 ± 0.2, and 5.0 ± 0.0, respectively. The subjective PET image quality score in the G2 group was significantly higher than that of the conventional digital PET/CT with full-dose ^{18}F-FDG group, which was 3.7 ± 0.6. Furthermore, it was observed that the liver SNR in G2 (11.7 ± 1.5) was considerably higher compared with that in the conventional digital PET/CT group (8.3 ± 1.2). In G2, the average SUV_{max} and SUV_{mean} of the liver were 3.4 ± 0.5 and 2.7 ± 0.5, respectively. These values were significantly higher than those observed in the conventional digital PET/CT group (2.9 ± 0.5 and 2.1 ± 0.3, respectively; $p < 0.001$). Additionally, the average SUV_{max} and SUV_{mean} of the blood pool in G2 were 2.5 ± 0.5 and 2.0 ± 0.4, respectively. These values were significantly higher than those of the conventional digital PET/CT group (2.2 ± 0.4 and 1.5 ± 0.2, respectively)

($p < 0.05$). While the mean and SD value of SUV_{max} of the lesions and the target-to-background ratio (TBR) were not notably different between G2 (9.2 ± 7.8, 4.7 ± 3.9) and the conventional digital PET/CT group (8.1 ± 5.7, 5.4 ± 3.9). All lesions could be detected in the G2 and G4 groups when using G15 as a reference.

In comparison to conventional digital PET/CT imaging, the results indicated that the TB PET/CT half-dose (1.85 MBq/kg) ^{18}F-FDG image, reconstructed in just 2 min, could meet the requirements for clinical diagnostic imaging. Furthermore, its image quality was better than that of conventional PET/CT utilizing the clinical routine full-dose ^{18}F-FDG for lung cancer (Fig. 6.1).

6.1.2 Comparative Study of Half-Dose and Full-Dose TB PET/CT Imaging

The $SNR = k\sqrt{S \times A \times T}$ formula comprises k as a constant, S as the number of detection events and sensitivity, A as the radiopharmaceutical activity, and T as the scan time [4]. While k and S are the fixed values for a given instrument, maintaining a consistent SNR requires an inversely proportional relationship between A and T. To evaluate the feasibility and reliability of half-dose ^{18}F-FDG PET imaging, our team conducted a comparison between half-dose ^{18}F-FDG TB PET/CT and full-dose TB PET/CT imaging [5]. We selected 50 patients with colorectal cancer who underwent half-dose ^{18}F-FDG TB PET/CT before treatment, and another 50 patients with colorectal cancer who underwent full-dose (3.70 MBq/kg) ^{18}F-FDG TB PET/CT before surgery, from our database. Both groups were matched for information such as patient age, sex, BMI, history of diabetes, waiting time after injection, pathological type of intestinal cancer, and lesion size. We compared and analyzed the ^{18}F-FDG PET images from the half-dose and full-dose groups.

The TB PET acquisition time for the half-dose group was 15 min (G15). The data was then reconstructed by cutting the data into 1 min, 2 min, 3 min, 4 min, and 10 min, and these images were labeled as G1, G2, G3, G4, and G10, respectively. By contrast, the full-dose group had a PET acquisition time of 5 min (G5′) and was reconstructed with data cut into 30 s, 1 min, and 2 min,

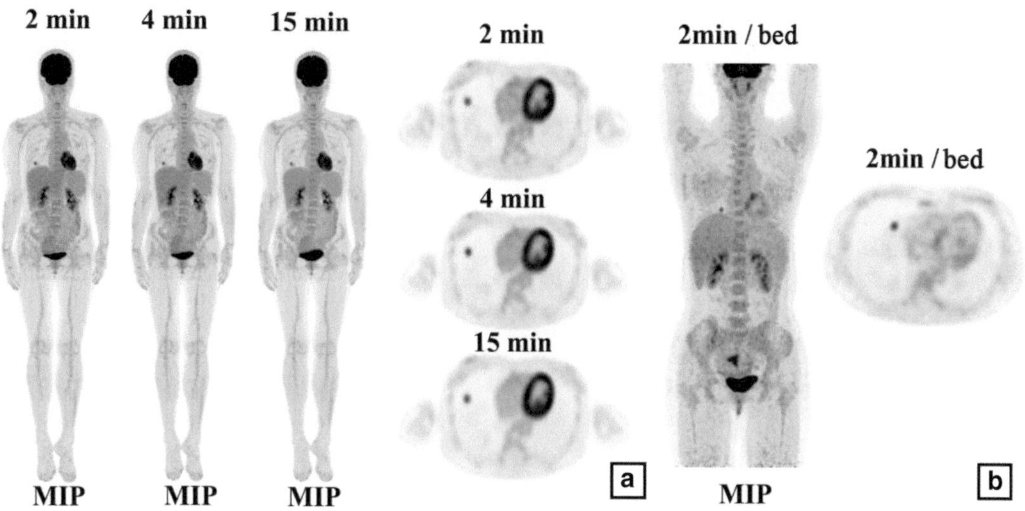

Fig. 6.1 Half-dose ^{18}F-FDG TB PET with acquisition time of 2 min presents image quality comparable to that of conventional full-dose digital PET images. (**a**) A 51-year-old female patient with invasive adenocarcinoma (grade II–III) in the lower lobe of the right lung. Maximum density projection (MIP) and cross-sectional images of half-dose ^{18}F-FDG TB PET images acquired for 2 min, 4 min, and 15 min. (**b**) A 43-year-old female patient with adenocarcinoma (grade II–III) in the middle lobe of the right lung. MIP and cross-sectional images of conventional digital PET with full-dose of ^{18}F-FDG acquired at a speed of 2 min/bed

resulting in images labeled G0.5′, G1′, and G2′. The image reconstruction conditions used were the same as in the first part of this section.

Both subjective and objective indicators were used to evaluate PET image quality. The subjective evaluation criteria and methods for PET image quality were consistent with those used in the previous section. Additionally, semi-quantitative indicators for image quality were assessed objectively, including SUV_{max}, SUV_{mean}, and SNR in areas such as the liver, mediastinal blood, and muscle. To measure the background uptake values of the liver, the procedure involved outlining an ROI with a diameter of 20 mm in each of the upper right anterior lobe, lower right lobe, right posterior lobe, and left outer lobe of the liver. The average value of these measurements was used as a representative semi-quantitative measurement of the whole liver. This approach avoided all identifiable lesions and large intrahepatic vessels. Similarly, an ROI of 20 mm in diameter was also outlined at the level of the third sacral foramen in each of the bilateral gluteus maximus muscles. To represent the semi-quantitative measurement of the muscle, the average of values was calculated. The SNR was then obtained by dividing the mean standardized uptake value by its standard deviation (SD). Based on the formula $SNR = k\sqrt{S \times A \times T}$, objective semi-quantitative metrics and subjective scores were chosen to compare the PET images of the different groups, namely G1 with G0.5′, G2 with G1′, G4 with G2′, and G10 with G5′. The metrics chosen for objective analysis of lesions included SUV_{max} and the TBR. The SUVmax of lesions was measured using the volume of interest (VOI), while the TBR was calculated by dividing the SUV_{max} of the lesion by the SUV_{mean} of the liver. The detection rate of lesions was calculated using the PET images of G15 and G5′ as the reference for each group, respectively.

The subjective evaluation of image quality revealed that, in the half-dose group, the scores for G15, G10, G4, G3, G2, and G1 were 4.98 ± 0.10, 4.57 ± 0.25, 3.93 ± 0.23, 3.28 ± 0.43, 3.00 ± 0.20, and 2.06 ± 0.19, respectively. In the full-dose group, the scores for G5′, G2′, G1′, and G0.5′ were 4.47 ± 0.40, 3.92 ± 0.23, 2.95 ± 0.18, and 2.16 ± 0.34, respectively. The image quality scores for G3 and G2′ were ≥3, which met clinical diagnosis requirements. Objective evaluation of the images showed significantly lower liver SNR (13.48 ± 2.36), mediastinal blood pool SNR (16.94 ± 6.17), and muscle SNR (11.50 ± 2.60) for G3 than for G15 (30.11 ± 10.07 for liver SNR, 31.45 ± 11.55 for blood pool SNR, and 20.87 ± 9.02 for muscle; all $p < 0.001$). Colorectal lesions exhibited significantly higher SUV_{max} (23.3 ± 12.9) and TBR (8.9 ± 4.8) in G3 than in G15 (20.1 ± 11.0 and 7.8 ± 4.2, respectively; both $p < 0.05$). In contrast, for metastatic lymph nodes and liver lesions, neither SUV_{max} nor TBR of G3 was statistically different from that of G15 (both $p > 0.05$). In the half-dose group, the 56 colorectal lesions confirmed by surgical pathology were visible in all groups. The number of lymph nodes with increased glucose metabolism was 37 in G1, 38 in G2, and 39 in the remaining groups. One liver metastasis lesion was missed in both the G1 and G2 groups. The results of this study showed that compared with full-dose ^{18}F-FDG TB PET/CT, half-dose ^{18}F-FDG TB PET/CT can be used for the diagnosis and staging of colorectal cancer. Moreover, its image quality, with an acquisition time of 3 min, could meet the requirements for clinical diagnostic.

In conclusion, half-dose ^{18}F-FDG TB PET/CT can be used for the diagnosis and staging of colorectal cancer, and its image quality, with a 3-min acquisition time, can meet clinical diagnostic needs when compared with full-dose ^{18}F-FDG TB PET/CT. There was no significant difference in subjective and objective PET image quality between half-dose (Fig. 6.2) and full-dose (Fig. 6.3) TB PET/CT imaging in the comparisons between the G1 and G0.5′, G2 and G1′, G4 and G2′, and G10 and G5′ groups. This finding reinforces the feasibility and reliability of half-dose TB PET/CT imaging.

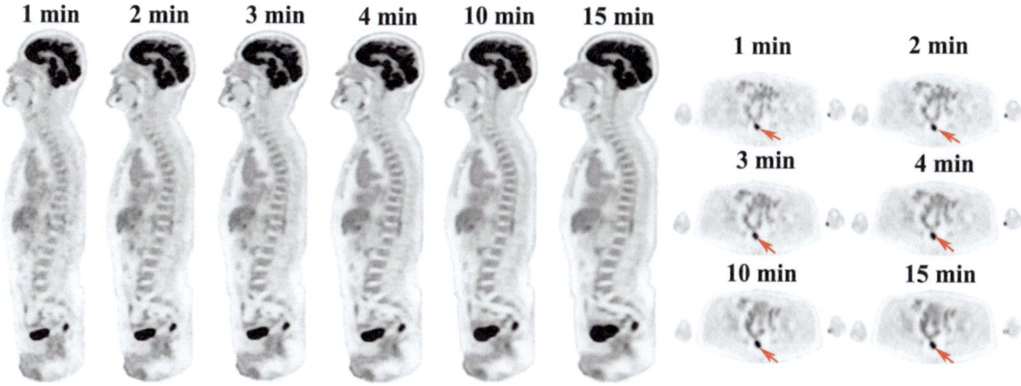

Fig. 6.2 Half-dose TB PET images of a patient with rectal cancer. A 79-year-old male patient with rectal ulcerative adenocarcinoma of grade II. The half-dose (3.4 mCi) ^{18}F-FDG TB PET images were acquired for 15 min and were divided into 1-min, 2-min, 3-min, 4-min, and 10-min images, respectively. These PET images show noise that gradually decreased with the increase of the acquisition time, and the quality of the reconstructed 1-min image was poor

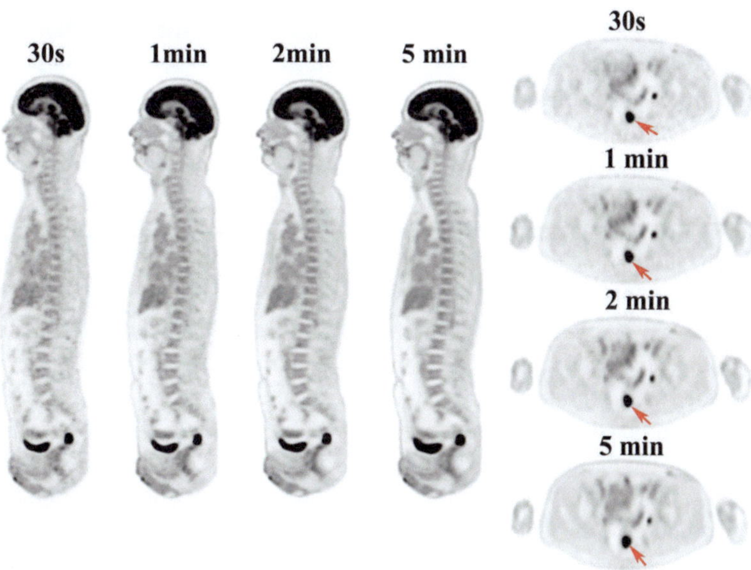

Fig. 6.3 Full-dose TB PET images of a patient with rectal cancer. A 54-year-old male patient with rectal ulcerative adenocarcinoma of grade II–III. Full-dose (6.2 mCi) ^{18}F-FDG TB PET/CT PET images were acquired for 5 min and were divided into 30-s, 1-min, and 2-min images, respectively. These PET images show noise that gradually decreased with the increase of acquisition time, and the quality of the reconstructed 30-s image was poor

6.2 Validation of Half-Dose TB PET/CT Acquisition Conditions

Image quality correlated positively with acquisition time at a constant injection dose. Suitable acquisition conditions for half-dose ^{18}F-FDG TB PET/CT in oncological imaging have been initially established; however, further validation and refinement are needed.

Patients undergoing half-dose ^{18}F-FDG TB PET/CT imaging at our center were retrospectively analyzed and divided into an initial exploratory cohort and a clinical validation cohort [6]. Forty-six oncology patients, including those with lung, colorectal, biliary, liver, and gastric tumors, underwent half-dose ^{18}F-FDG TB PET/CT imaging between October 2019 and December 2019. These patients were used as the exploratory cohort to establish the initial protocol for half-dose ^{18}F-FDG TB PET/CT imaging. The clinical validation cohort included 147 patients with malignancy or suspected malignancy between December 2019 and June 2021 to validate the results of the exploratory cohort and to further determine the optimal range of scan times. The ^{18}F-FDG dose to the patients was 1.88 ± 0.09 MBq/kg, and waiting time (injection and imaging intervals) was 64.7 ± 17.2 min. The initial exploration cohort had a PET image acquisition time of 15 min (G15), and the images were then reconstructed using the first 1 min, 2 min, 3 min, 5 min, and 8 min of data, which were abbreviated as G1, G2, G3, G5, and G8, respectively. In the validation cohort, images acquired using acquisition durations of 15 min and 10 min were collectively referred to as Gs images. To further explore the results of the exploration cohort, all PET images were reconstructed and further divided into G8, G5, G3, and G2 images. The image reconstruction conditions were as follows: OSEM algorithm incorporating high-resolution TOF and PSF modeling, 3 iterations, 20 subsets, matrix 192 × 192, slice thickness 1.443 mm, and Gaussian post-filter 3 mm.

The image quality was evaluated on both subjective and objective dimensions. Subjective image analysis was performed as in Sect. 6.1. The objective evaluation of PET image quality included the semi-quantitative parameters of the liver and mediastinal blood pool: SUV_{max}, SUV_{mean}, and SD. The same size of ROIs was outlined simultaneously on the same position in the same section of the image at different acquisition times to reduce inter-group differences. Objective analyses of lesions included SUV_{max}, peak SUV (SUV_{peak}), and TBR. Lesion SUV_{max} and SUV_{peak} were measured using the VOI. The TBR was calculated by dividing the lesion SUV_{max} by the liver SUV_{mean}. The number of lesions found in the G15 (exploration dataset) and Gs (validation dataset) images were selected as references to calculate lesion detection rates for images with different acquisition durations. Two nuclear medicine physicians analyzed the subjective image quality for each cohort, and lesion detection rates were evaluated at ≥2-week intervals after completion of the initial analysis.

The results of the study showed that the subjective image quality scores for G1, G2, G3, G5, and G8 in the exploration cohort were 2.0 ± 0.2, 2.9 ± 0.3, 3.0 ± 0.0, 3.9 ± 0.2 and 4.2 ± 0.4, respectively. Two cases in G1 had an image quality score of 1, while the subjective scores for the remaining groups were ≥2. The objective evaluation of PET image quality demonstrated a gradual decrease in image noise and a gradual increase in liver SNR with increasing acquisition time. The pathological results confirmed a total of 75 lesions in 46 cases. Using G15 as a reference, the lesion detection rates in G1 and G2 were 85.3% (58/68) and 97.1% (66/68), respectively, while in the remaining groups, the lesion detection rates were 100% (68/68).

A total of 147 cases were included in the validation cohort, including tumors from multiple sites throughout the body, of which a total of 240 lesions (163 primary tumors, 69 suspected lymph node metastases, and 8 distant metastases) were detected. The subjective image quality scores for G2, G3, G5, G8, and Gs were 3.0 ± 0.2, 3.0 ± 0.1, 3.6 ± 0.5, 4.0 ± 0.3, and 4.4 ± 0.5, respectively. The subjective scores for G2 and G3 were basically at the same level (approximately 3). A total of 204 lesions were detected in G15, with 100% (204/204), 99.0% (202/204), 94.1% (192/204), and 90.2% (184/204) of the lesions being detected in G8, G5, G3, and G2, respectively.

The results showed that an acquisition time of 2 min could obtain an image quality that met the clinical diagnostic requirements. For lung tumors, an acquisition time of 2 min by half-dose ^{18}F-FDG TB PET/CT was sufficient for clinical diagnostic needs, and was highly effective in lesion diagnostic performance (Fig. 6.4), while an acquisition time of 3–5 min was adequate for most clinical applications, such as gastrointestinal tumors (Fig. 6.5). For diseases of the hepatobiliary system, an acquisition time of 5–8 min is more conducive to obtaining adequate diagnostic or evaluation information (Fig. 6.6). In summary, the 8-min acquisition protocol provides high-quality PET images and is an alternative to the 10-min protocol with respect to lesion detectability.

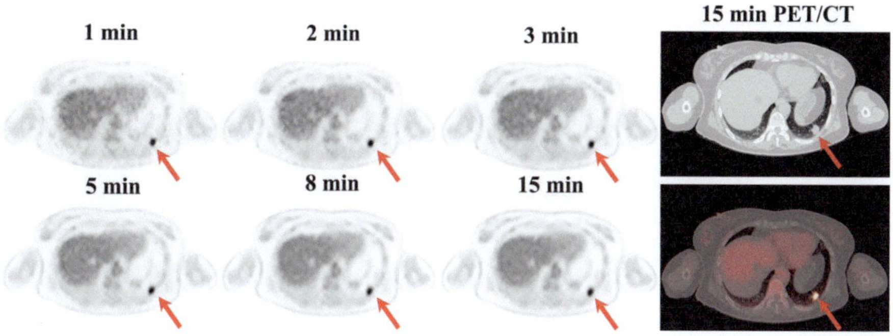

Fig. 6.4 Half-dose TB PET/CT images of a patients with lung cancer. A 60-year-old female patient with suspected lung cancer. Half-dose ^{18}F-FDG TB PET/CT image was reconstructed into 1-min, 2-min, 3-min, 5-min, 8-min, and 15-min transverse PET images, CT image, and 15-min fused PET/CT image. As shown by the red arrows, the lesion in the lower lobe of the left lung shows high glucose metabolism and is visible on images of different acquisition times. The liver SNR of the reconstructed 1-min PET image was poor. It was pathologically confirmed to be a poorly-differentiated acinar-predominant adenocarcinoma with a small proportion of micropapillary type

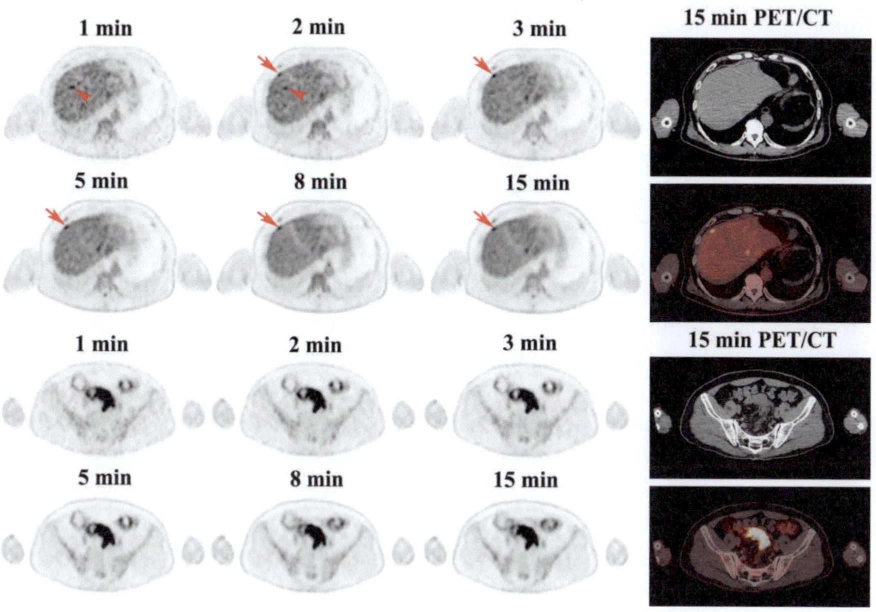

Fig. 6.5 Half-dose TB PET/CT images of a patient with sigmoid colon cancer and liver metastases. A 56-year-old male patient with suspected liver metastasis from sigmoid colon cancer. Half-dose ^{18}F-FDG TB PET/CT imaging was reconstructed into 1-min, 2-min, 3-min, 5-min, 8-min, and 15-min transverse PET images, CT image, and 15-min PET/CT fused image. Liver metastasis can be demonstrated on the 2-min, 3-min, 5-min, 8-min, and 15-min PET images (as indicated by red arrows); however, the 1-min PET image cannot identify the lesion from the background noise. Postoperative pathology confirmed poorly-differentiated ulcerated adenocarcinoma of the sigmoid colon with liver metastasis

As the BMI increases, the number of photons emitted out of the body decreases because of increased photon attenuation and scattering rate, and the peak noise equivalent count rate (NECR) decreases, reducing the quality of the PET image, provided that the injected dose remains constant. There were 193 patients in the two cohorts, including 23 cases with BMI ≥28 and 170 cases

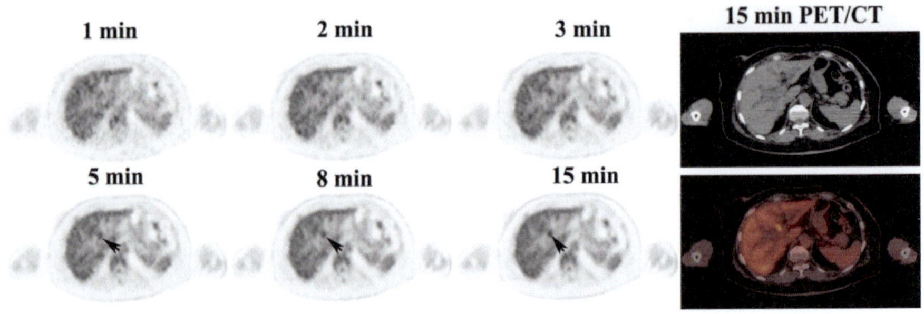

Fig. 6.6 Half-dose TB PET/CT images of a patient with cholangiocarcinoma at the hepatic hilar. A 67-year-old female patient with suspected cholangiocarcinoma at the hepatic hilar. Half-dose ^{18}F-FDG TB PET/CT imaging was reconstructed into 1-min, 2-min, 3-min, 5-min, 8-min, and 15-min transverse PET images, CT image, and 15-min fused PET/CT image. The lesion (black arrows) is visible on the 5-min, 8-min, and 15-min PET images, while the 3-min PET image fails to show the lesion. The postoperative pathological diagnosis was grade-III cholangiocarcinoma at the hepatic hilar with infiltration of the entire bile duct wall and involvement to adjacent liver tissue

with BMI <28. The subjective PET image quality scores for G2, G3, G5, G8, and Gs (acquisition time, 10 or 15 min) were 2.5 ± 0.6, 2.9 ± 0.3, 3.1 ± 0.3, 3.7 ± 0.4, and 4.2 ± 0.4 for patients with BMI ≥28, respectively, with mean scores slightly lower than those for patients with BMI <28, whose corresponding subjective scores for G2, G3, G5, G8, and Gs were 2.7 ± 0.5, 3.0 ± 0.2, 3.5 ± 0.5, 3.9 ± 0.2, and 4.2 ± 0.2, respectively. The differences in subjective PET image quality scores between G2 and G3 with BMI ≥28 and BMI <28 were not significant (p = 0.14, p = 0.179), whereas the differences in subjective scores between G5, G8, and Gs with BMI ≥28 and BMI <28 were statistically significant (p = 0.000, p = 0.04, p = 0.004). Therefore, the acquisition time for patients with BMI ≥28 should be prolonged to more than 5 min to obtain better image quality when using half-dose ^{18}F-FDG TB PET/CT imaging in clinical practice.

6.3 Application of Half-Dose Total-Body PET/CT Imaging in Takayasu's Arteritis

Active Takayasu's arteritis (TA) is characterized by the infiltration of inflammatory cells in the affected vascular wall. PET/CT imaging is used to detect this condition, showing a notable accumulation of ^{18}F-FDG. This imaging method is highly sensitive in identifying active inflammatory lesions and serves as a useful adjunct to laboratory and other diagnostic tests. However, the identification of vascular wall inflammatory lesions can be affected by several factors, including high levels of ^{18}F-FDG concentration in the blood that might mask the lesions. To address this issue, TB PET/CT is preferred [7, 8]. TB PET/CT involves acquiring images at 2 h after the injection of half-dose ^{18}F-FDG, reducing the specific activity of ^{18}F-FDG in the blood because of the injection dose, attenuation, and excretion, and at the same time, allowing the lesions to fully take up the imaging agent for a longer time, thereby maximizing the contrast between the lesions and the blood background [6, 9]. Moreover, TB PET/CT offers total-body imaging, enabling easy identification of lower limb vascular lesions that might be missed during routine PET/CT examination (as shown in Fig. 6.7).

Our study involved 55 patients diagnosed with Takayasu's arteritis [10], in accordance with NIH criteria. These individuals received 2 h and 5 h half-dose TB PET/CT scans, with an injection of ^{18}F-FDG (1.85 MBq/kg). The images were reconstructed via ordered subset expectation maximization, with the use of the following conditions: 3 iterations, 20 subsets, a matrix size of 192 × 192, layer thickness of 1.443 mm, Gaussian filtering of 3 mm, time of flight, and point spread function. The classification of active and inactive Takayasu's arteritis was based on the 1990 standard set by the American College of Rheumatology

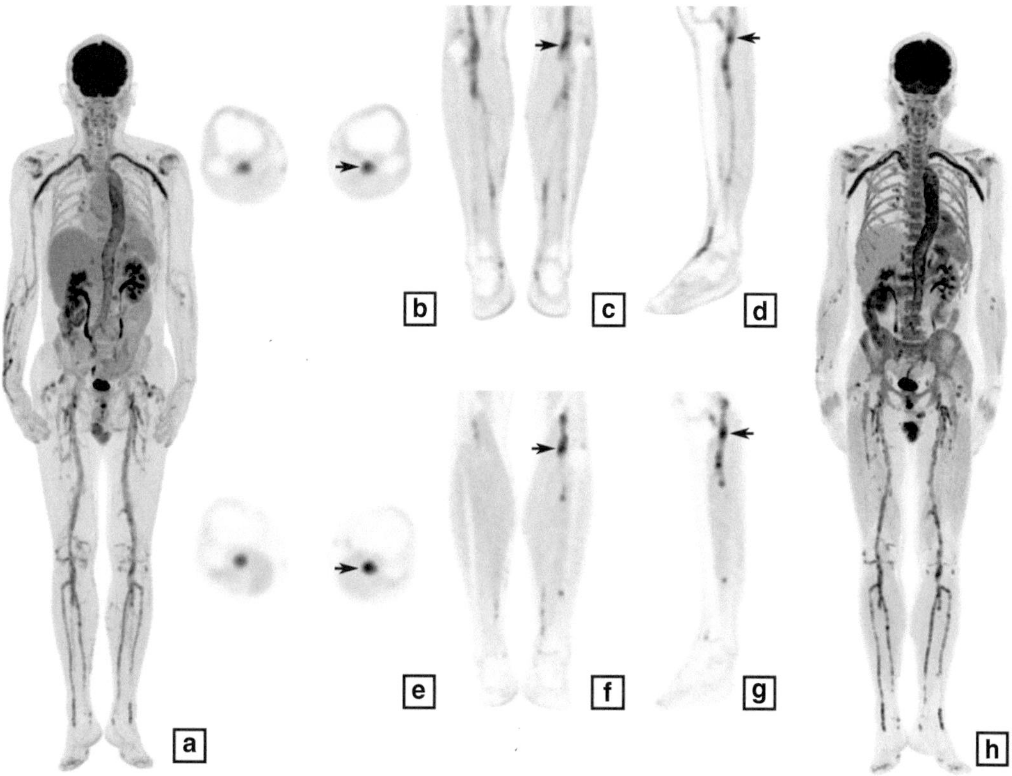

Fig. 6.7 Half-dose ^{18}F-FDG TB PET/CT imaging of a patient with giant cell arteritis. A 65-year-old male patient was diagnosed with giant cell arteritis. Half-dose ^{18}F-FDG TB PET imaging: (**a**) whole-body maximum intensity projection (MIP) of PET image 2 h post tracer administration, present the liver SUV_{max} (SUV_L) of 2.47 and the blood pool SUV_{max} (SUV_B) of 1.58; (**b–d**) Transverse, coronal, and sagittal PET images acquired 2 h post tracer injection, demonstrate a popliteal artery lesion; (**h**) MIP of PET image acquired at 5 h post injection present the SUV_L of 1.77 and the SUV_B of 0.44; (**e–h**) Cross-sectional, coronal, and sagittal PET images scanned 5 h post injection show that the popliteal artery lesion is more clear. In the 2-h and 5-h PET images, the SUV_{max} values of the popliteal artery lesion (arrows) were 4.77 and 6.55, respectively

(ACR). Among 55 patients, 39 had active disease active, and 16 had inactive disease. The uptake by vascular lesions was graded according to the three-grade method (I, II, III). In level I, the SUV_{max} of the lesions was lower than that of the liver. In level II, the SUV_{max} of the lesions was close to that of the liver. In level III, the SUV_{max} of the lesions was higher than that of the liver. Level II and III were considered as positive lesions. The aorta and its primary branches were divided into 26 segments, including the left and right common carotid artery, the left and right subclavian artery, the left and right pulmonary artery, the left and right renal artery, the left and right common iliac artery, the left and right femoral artery, the left and right popliteal artery, the left and right anterior tibial artery, and the left and right posterior tibial artery. The head and arm trunk, ascending aorta, aortic arch, pulmonary trunk, thoracic aorta, abdominal aorta, celiac trunk, and superior mesenteric artery were also included. If multiple lesions were present in one segment, only the lesion with the highest SUV_{max} was selected to represent the whole segment. The lesion-to-blood ratio (LBR) between the lesion and the blood pool was analyzed by calculating the lesion SUV_{max} value divided by the blood SUV_{max} value.

The half-dose ^{18}F-FDG TB PET/CT 2 h imaging demonstrated a lower blood pool background and better lesion contrast, as shown in Fig. 6.8. The high sensitivity of TB PET/CT, coupled with

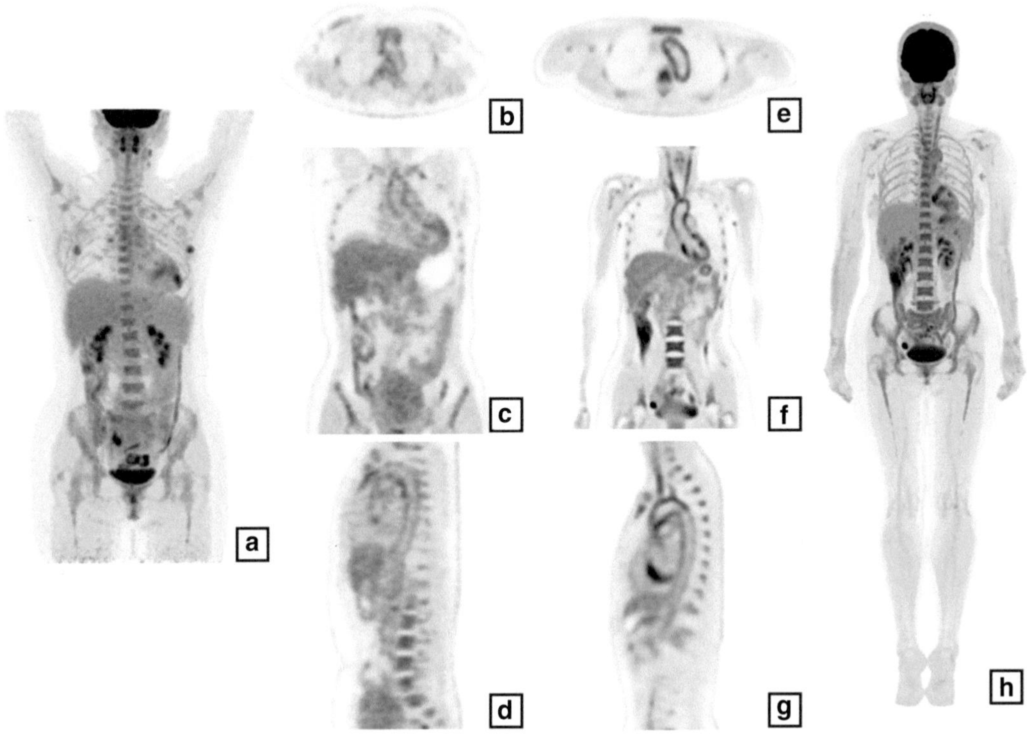

Fig. 6.8 Comparison between conventional ^{18}F-FDG PET/CT imaging and half-dose TB ^{18}F-FDG PET/CT imaging. (**a**–**d**) A 35-year-old female patient was diagnosed with active Takayasu's arteritis. The elevated erythrocyte sedimentation rate (ESR) was 52 mm/H, while the C-reactive protein (CRP) was normal. (**a**) Maximum intensity projection (MIP) of conventional ^{18}F-FDG PET acquired 2 h post-tracer injection reveals the liver SUV_{max} (SUV_L) of 2.35 and the SUV_{max} of blood pool (SUV_B) of 0.9; (**b**–**d**) Transverse, coronal, and sagittal PET images shows that the aorta can be seen on the PET images. (**e**–**h**) A 39-year-old female patient was diagnosed with active Takayasu's arteritis. The ESR and CRP were elevated, which were 43 mm/H and 17.9 mg/L, respectively. (**h**) MIP image of ^{18}F-FDG TB PET acquired 2 h after tracer injection reveals the SUV_L and SUV_B to be 1.99 and 0.7, respectively; (**e**–**g**) Transverse, coronal, and sagittal PET images shows that the aorta can be easily seen on the PET images. When comparing the image contrast between (**a**–**d**) and (**e**–**h**), it is easy to find that the background metabolism in the blood pool of the half-dose TB PET image is lower, and the vascular wall lesions are better displayed

15 min/bed acquisition, further improved the detection efficiency. The results indicated that lesions with the lowest uptake had a SUV_{max} of only 1.20, and an LBR of 2.22, highlighting the advantages of high sensitivity in TB PET/CT. Approximately 10% of Takayasu's arteritis lesions occur in the popliteal artery and the vessels below and can be easily missed by conventional PET/CT. However, with its long axial field of view, TB PET/CT can identify vascular lesions in the lower limbs that are often overlooked in routine examinations [7].

A study conducted in our center examined the efficacy of half-dose ^{18}F-FDG TB PET/CT 5 h imaging in detecting lesions of Takayasu's arteritis [11]. The study included 39 patients with active Takayasu's arteritis, resulting in 415 positive lesions being identified. The detection rates of active Takayasu's arteritis were 92.0% (382/415) and 94.2% (391/415), for 2 h and 5 h imaging, respectively, with the LBR being 3.67 and 7.59, respectively. In addition, 19 patients with inactive Takayasu's arteritis were examined, revealing 143 active lesions. The detection rates of the lesions were 97.9% (140/143) and 98.6% (141/143), for 2 h and 5 h imaging, respectively, with the LBR being 2.99 and 5.71, respectively. The results indicate that half-dose ^{18}F-FDG TB PET/CT 5 h imaging can improve the detection efficiency for lesions of Takayasu's

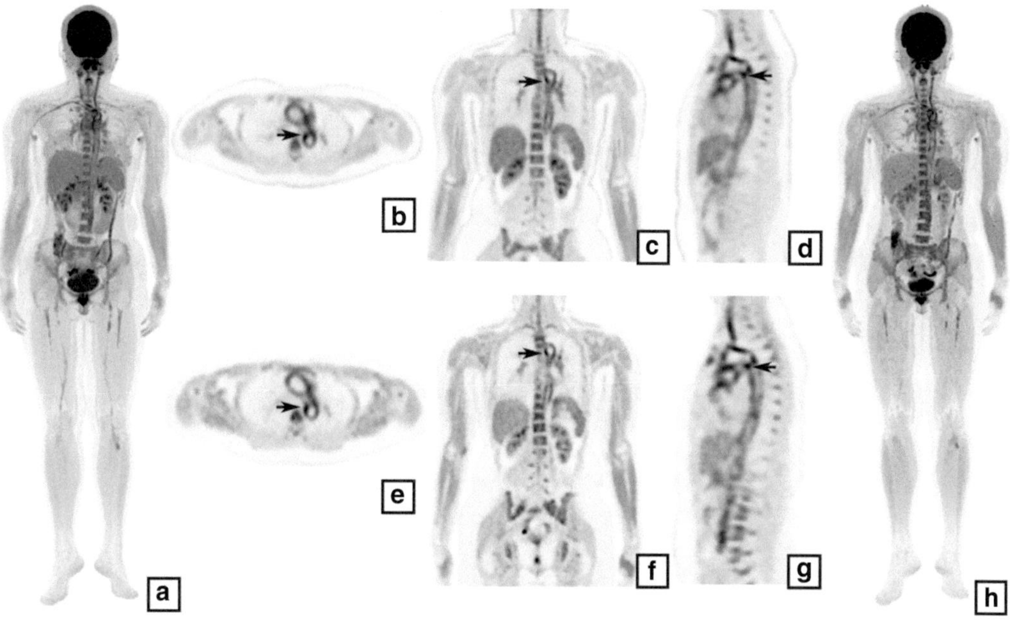

Fig. 6.9 Half-dose ^{18}F-FDG TB PET/CT imaging in patients with active Takayasu's arteritis. A 21-year-old female was diagnosed with active Takayasu's arteritis. Half-dose ^{18}F-FDG TB PET/CT imaging: (**a**) Whole-body MIP of PET image acquired 2 h after tracer injection reveals the liver SUV_{max} (SUV_L) and the SUV_{max} of blood pool (SUV_B) to be 2.46 and 0.98, respectively; (**b**–**d**) Corresponding transverse, coronal, and sagittal PET images demonstrated thoracic aortic lesions; (**h**) Whole-body MIP of PET image acquired 5 h after tracer injection reveals the SUV_L and SUV_B to be 2.04 and 0.48, respectively; (**e**–**g**) Corresponding transverse, coronal, and sagittal PET images shows the thoracic aortic lesions with better image contrast. In the 2-h and 5-h images, the SUV_{max} of the active TA lesions in the thoracic aorta (arrows) were 6.56 and 7.62, respectively

arteritis. The average LBR of lesions in the 5 h imaging was higher and the contrast was increased compared with those in the 2 h imaging, as shown in Fig. 6.9. However, both 2 h and 5 h imaging missed some lesions. Therefore, 5 h imaging and 2 h imaging should complement each other. Depending on the clinical needs, a combined approach for 5 h imaging and 2 h imaging could improve the lesion detection efficiency.

References

1. Filippi L, Schillaci O. Total-body [^{18}F] FDG PET/CT scan has stepped into the arena: the faster, the better. Is it always true. Eur J Nucl Med Mol Imaging. 2022;49(10):3322–7.
2. Boellaard R, Delgado-Bolton R, Oyen WJ, et al. FDG PET/CT: EANM procedure guidelines for tumour imaging: version 2.0. Eur J Nucl Med Mol Imaging. 2015;42(2):328–54.
3. Tan H, Sui X, Yin H, et al. Total-body PET/CT using half-dose FDG and compared with conventional PET/CT using full-dose FDG in lung cancer. Eur J Nucl Med Mol Imaging. 2021;48(6):1966–75.
4. Cherry SR, Jones T, Karp JS, et al. Total-body PET: maximizing sensitivity to create new opportunities for clinical research and patient care. J Nucl Med. 2018;59(1):3–12.
5. Tan H, Mao W, Cao Y, et al. Half-dose versus full-dose ^{18}F-FDG total-body PET/CT in patients with colorectal cancer. Nucl Med Commun. 2022;43(8):928–36.
6. He Y, Gu Y, Yu H, et al. Optimizing acquisition times for total-body positron emission tomography/computed tomography with half-dose ^{18}F-fluorodeoxyglucose in oncology patients. EJNMMI Phys. 2022;9(1):45.
7. Derlin T, Spencer BA, Mamach M, et al. Exploring vessel wall biology in vivo by ultrasensitive total-body PET. J Nucl Med. 2023;64(3):416–22.
8. Kubota K, Itoh M, Ozaki K, et al. Advantage of delayed whole-body FDG-PET imaging for tumour detection. Eur J Nucl Med. 2001;28(6):696–703.
9. Chen W, Liu L, Li Y, et al. Evaluation of pediatric malignancies using total-body PET/CT with half-dose [^{18}F]-FDG. Eur J Nucl Med Mol Imaging. 2022;49(12):4145–55.

10. Cai D, Adili D, Shi H. Value of ^{18}F-FDG total-body PET/CT 2-hour imaging in detection of Takayasu arteritis. Chin J Nucl Med Mol Imaging. 2022;42(8):462–6.
11. Adili D, Cai D, Wu B, et al. An exploration of the feasibility and clinical value of half-dose 5-h total-body ^{18}F-FDG PET/CT scan in patients with Takayasu arteritis. Eur J Nucl Med Mol Imaging. 2023;50(8):2375–85. https://doi.org/10.1007/s00259-023-06168-6.

7 Clinical Application of Extra Low-Dose Total-Body PET/CT Scan

Yan Hu, Ha Wu, Huaping Gao, and Hongcheng Shi

According to the corresponding principles or guidelines, the radiation dose received by patients should be in the safe range during nuclear medicine diagnosis and treatment. Radiation can cause deterministic or random effects on the human body. However, dose optimization helps to reduce the radiation exposure of patients and staff in the clinic. Dose optimization should follow the principle of "As low as reasonably achievable" (ALARA), i.e., reducing the injection activity of the imaging agent as much as possible on the premise that the image quality meets the needs of clinical diagnosis [1]. The radiation dose of positron emission tomography–computed tomography (PET/CT) scanning comes from two aspects: X-ray radiation from CT and β-ray and γ-ray radiation from PET. X-rays have high energy and strong ionization effects, which can induce various biological effects in the human body and account for the majority of the PET/CT radiation dose. Reduction of the CT radiation dose can be achieved by reducing the tube current and tube voltage, increasing the pitch, diminishing noise filtering, or adopting new reconstruction algorithms. The radiation dose of PET originates from the β-rays emitted by the imaging agent injected into the body and the γ-rays released by annihilation radiation, which correlates positively with the activity of the injected imaging agent.

Radiation exposure caused by radioactive tracer during PET imaging has been a great concern. The radiation dose of a conventional whole-body PET/CT imaging is about 7–10 mSv [2]. The guidelines for pediatric ^{118}F-fluorodeoxyglucose (FDG) PET/CT imaging emphasize that the radiation dose should be reduced as much as possible on the premise of image quality meeting the diagnostic requirements [3]. The radiation dose of ^{18}F-FDG PET/CT imaging is reduced to 0.4 mSv with 1/10 of the recommended injected activity (3.7 MBq/kg) in the guidelines, which is important for radiation sensitive populations, such as infants, children, and adolescents, and also has obvious advantages for patients who need multiple PET/CT imaging in a short time.

The axial field of view of conventional PET/CT is 15–30 cm. Subject to its sensitivity, reducing the activity of imaging agent injection will lead to insufficient counting, increased image noise, reduced image quality, and a decreased lesion detection rate. To reduce the injection activity of the imaging agent, it is necessary to increase the acquisition time to effectively avoid the degradation of image quality caused by insufficient counting. However, for children with low compliance or severely ill patients with poor tolerance, excessive acquisition time will increase their discomfort, generate motion artifacts during the examination, and thus reduce the image quality. The total-body PET/CT (TB PET/CT)

Y. Hu · H. Wu · H. Gao · H. Shi (✉)
Department of Nuclear Medicine, Zhongshan Hospital, Fudan University, Shanghai, China
e-mail: shi.hongcheng@zs-hospital.sh.cn

© Shanghai Scientific and Technical Publishers 2024
H. Shi et al. (eds.), *Total-Body PET/CT*, https://doi.org/10.1007/978-981-97-5065-8_7

with an axial field of 194 cm has more than 400,000 lutetium silicate scintillation crystals, greatly improving the photon detection efficiency, which is 40-fold higher than that of conventional PET/CT, making low-activity PET imaging possible [4, 5]. It has been reported that TB PET/CT imaging still shows an excellent performance when the injection activity was reduced to 1/20 of the recommended standard activity. The radiation dose was significantly reduced and the image signal-to-noise ratio increased about 6.9 times compared with those of conventional PET/CT [6]. The TB PET/CT imaging with 1/10 injected activity has obvious advantages; however, it has not been widely used in clinical practice, and its methodological connotation and clinical application value would benefit from wider publicity.

7.1 Methodology for TB PET/CT Imaging with 1/10 Activity ^{18}F-FDG

Taking the injection activity (3.7 MBq/kg) recommended by the European Association of Nuclear Medicine (EANM) for conventional PET/CT as a reference, our team defined 1/10 of the recommended activity as an ultra-low activity (0.37 MBq/kg).

The injected activity and the appropriate acquisition time required to obtain the PET image quality that meets the diagnostic requirements were determined. Based on this, 1/10 activity TB PET/CT imaging was performed on a group of patients with tumors, and the acquisition time to meet the diagnostic needs was optimized through the evaluation of PET image quality simulating different acquisition times.

Thirty patients with pathologically confirmed malignant tumors who met the criteria of fasting blood glucose <7.0 mmol/L and body mass index (BMI) <30 kg/m^2 were enrolled. All patients underwent 1/10 activity (0.37 MBq/kg) TB PET/CT imaging. There were 20 men and 10 women, with a mean age of 66.10 ± 8.44 years, a mean BMI of 22.73 ± 3.28 kg/m^2, an average of fasting blood glucose level of 5.75 ± 0.66 mmol/L, a mean injection activity of 25.53 ± 4.07 MBq, and the mean uptake time post injection was 60.97 ± 5.96 min. Based on the principle of wide coverage, the 30 patients with cancer included 1 case of laryngeal cancer, 1 case of lung cancer, 2 cases of esophageal cancer, 1 case of mediastinal sarcoma, 4 cases of liver cancer, 3 cases of pancreatic cancer, 11 cases of colorectal cancer, 4 cases of bladder cancer, 2 cases of ovarian cancer, and 1 case of lymphoma.

The PET image acquisition time of all patients was 15 min. Then, the first 1 min, 2 min, 4 min, 8 min, 10 min, and 15 min of the raw data were reconstructed to simulate the faster acquisition at different times, referred to as G1, G2, G4, G8, G10, and G15, respectively. PET reconstructions adopted ordered subset expectation maximization (OSEM) iterative algorithm. Time of flight (TOF) and point spread function (PSF) were added to improve the spatial resolution of the PET images. The reconstruction parameters were as follows: 3 iterations, 20 subsets, matrix of 192 × 192, slice thickness of 1.443 mm, and a full width at half maximum of the Gaussian filter function of 3 mm.

PET imaging diagnosis is mainly based on the subjective judgment of nuclear medicine physicians, together with certain objective semi-quantitative analysis indicators. In this study, the image quality evaluation was carried out from two dimensions: subjective assessment and objective evaluation.

The PET image quality was evaluated independently by two experienced nuclear medicine physicians. The qualitative analysis of image quality was scored on a scale of 1–5.1, unacceptable image quality: extremely poor contrast with significant noise; 2, poor image quality: low contrast with noise; 3, acceptable image quality: moderate contrast with noise; 4, good image quality: good contrast with less noise; 5, excellent image quality: perfect contrast with minimal noise. A score of 3 represented the minimum acceptable image quality.

To avoid the impact of anthropic factors on the image quality evaluation as far as possible, two raters were assigned to evaluate the PET image quality in a blind manner according to the random principle, and the process was repeated after an interval of more than 1 week. The final score was determined using the average score of the two raters. The intra-observer and inter-observer agreement for the qualitative scores were analyzed (0.00–0.20, low; 0.21–0.40, medium; 0.41–0.60, moderate; 0.61–0.80, good; 0.81–1.00, excellent).

Semi-quantitative analysis is a method in which nuclear medicine physicians draw a region of interest (ROI) on the image (concealing the patients' basic information) and then acquire information to obtain semi-quantitative analysis indicators. To obtain the normal liver semi-quantitative analysis indicators, an ROI with a diameter of 2 cm was delineated where the portal vein bifurcated at the right lobe level of the liver and at least 1 cm away from the liver edge. In addition, the influence of the lesion should be avoided when drawing the ROI. To obtain the semi-quantitative analysis indicators of the lesion, the ROI adapted to the lesion size was drawn on the corresponding PET transverse slice with the maximum diameter in the CT image. Semi-quantitative parameters of PET images included: the maximum standard uptake value (SUV_{max}), the mean standard uptake value (SUV_{mean}), and the standard deviation (SD). Liver SUV_{max}, liver SUV_{mean}, liver SD, and lesion SUV_{max} were measured and recorded, respectively. The liver signal-to-noise ratio (SNR) was calculated by dividing the SUV_{mean} by its SD, and the target-to-background ratio (TBR) was calculated by dividing the lesion SUV_{max} by the liver SUV_{max}.

The subjective evaluation demonstrated that the image quality score achieved good intra-observer and inter-observer agreements at different acquisition times (Table 7.1). With the extension of acquisition time, the intra-observer and inter-observer agreements for the 8 min, 10 min, and 15 min images gradually increased. The image quality at 1 min and 2 min was poor, and could not meet the needs of clinical diagnosis. When the acquisition time was 4 min, the image quality score was close to 3. When the acquisition time was more than 8 min, the image quality score was greater than 3, and the image quality score reached 5 at 15 min.

The subjective evaluation of the image quality with 1/10 activity allowed us to conclude that the image quality acquired over 8 min was equivalent to that at 15 min.

The objective analysis of PET semi-quantitative parameters showed that the lesion SUV_{max} increased with the extension of acquisition time, and the increase trend slowed down when the uptake of lesion reached a certain level (Table 7.2). The liver SUV_{max} decreased continuously with the increase in acquisition time, indicating that the longer the acquisition time, the lower the liver background. When the acquisition time was longer than 4 min, the declining trend of the liver background gradually became weaker. The TBR increased with the extension of acquisition time, but was slower at 4 min; no significant difference was found between G4–G10 and G15.

Similar to the liver SUV_{max}, the liver SUV_{mean} and liver SD decreased gradually as the extension of acquisition time. There were obvious differences in liver SD between G1–G4 and G15, and the liver SD at 8 min was similar to that at 15 min. The SNR increased significantly with longer acquisition time, and the increased trend at 8 min was obvious. Statistical analysis showed that the

Table 7.1 Subjective analysis of image quality

Acquisition time (min)	Observer 1	Observer 2	Inter-kappa-value	Inter-kappa-value
1	1.10 ± 0.31	1.14 ± 0.35	0.898	0.849
2	2.07 ± 0.37	2.10 ± 0.41	0.902	0.885
4	3.00 ± 0.38	2.90 ± 0.49	0.895	0.750
8	4.07 ± 0.53	3.97 ± 0.63	0.900	0.852
10	4.38 ± 0.49	4.38 ± 0.49	0.921	0.854
15	4.62 ± 0.49	4.59 ± 0.50	0.945	0.930

This table was adapted with permission from a published JNM article [7]

Table 7.2 Semi-quantitative analysis parameters of PET image quality

Acquisition time (min)	Lesion SUV_{max}	Liver SUV_{max}	TBR	Liver SUV_{mean}	Liver SD	SNR
1	12.44 ± 5.00	4.56 ± 0.86	2.84 ± 1.36	2.80 ± 0.48	0.56 ± 0.19	5.41 ± 1.53
2	14.58 ± 6.86	3.80 ± 0.60	3.89 ± 1.80	2.78 ± 0.44	0.38 ± 0.11	7.67 ± 1.88
4	16.95 ± 7.78	3.53 ± 0.52	4.83 ± 2.18	2.77 ± 0.43	0.28 ± 0.08	10.41 ± 2.54
8	18.09 ± 8.26	3.31 ± 0.50	5.53 ± 2.50	2.73 ± 0.38	0.21 ± 0.06	13.46 ± 3.13
10	18.37 ± 8.06	3.21 ± 0.46	5.78 ± 2.50	2.72 ± 0.39	0.19 ± 0.06	14.72 ± 3.46
15	18.96 ± 7.93	3.08 ± 0.42	6.18 ± 2.52	2.70 ± 0.38	0.18 ± 0.05	15.65 ± 3.64

This table was adapted with permission from a published JNM article [7]

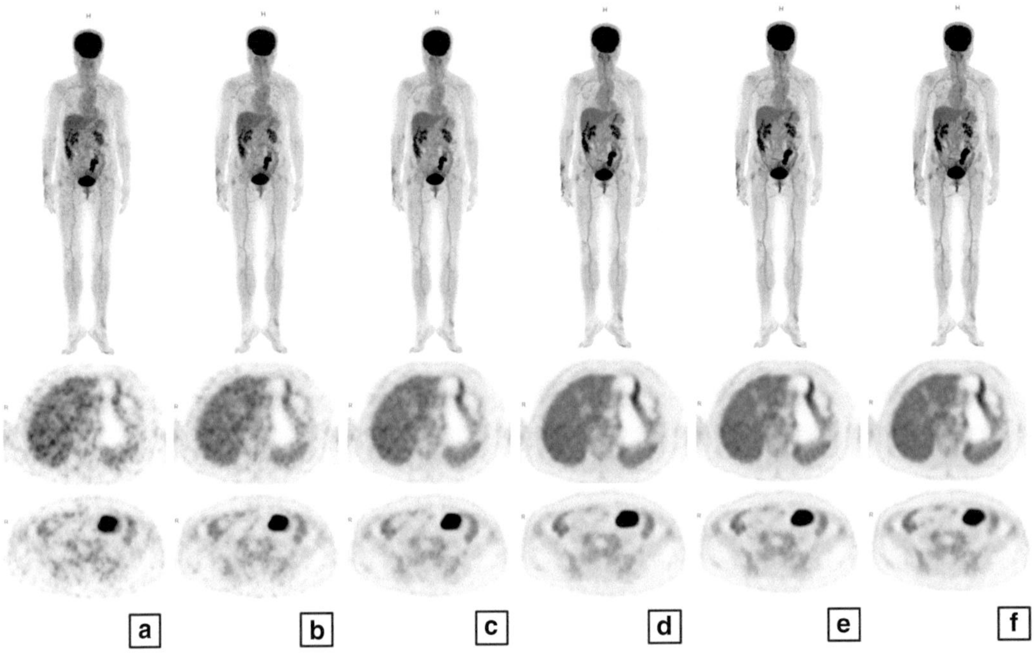

Fig. 7.1 The image quality of 1/10 activity TB PET acquired for 8 min was equivalent to those acquired for 15 min. PET images of a 70-year-old woman with sigmoid adenocarcinoma (grade II–III). Coronal PET images of the whole body, transverse view of the liver, and transverse view of the lesion (**a**–**f**) are shown for G1, G2, G4, G8, G10, and G15 reconstructions. The image quality of G8 was comparable to that of G10 and G15, and a superior image quality was observed in G8 than that in G1 and G2

SNR at 8 min was not significantly different from that at 15 min.

The subjective evaluation of image quality and the comprehensive analysis of semi-quantitative parameters allowed us to make the following conclusions: The image quality of 1/10 activity PET imaging with 8 min acquisition can meet the requirements for clinical diagnosis, and the lesion SUV_{max}, TBR, and SNR are not significantly different from those of PET imaging acquired in 15 min. These results preliminarily proved the clinical feasibility of 1/10 activity of ^{18}F-FDG TB PET/CT imaging (Fig. 7.1).

7.2 Clinical Validation of TB PET/CT Imaging with 1/10 Activity ^{18}F-FDG

Based on the previous analysis of the image quality of 1/10 activity ^{18}F-FDG TB PET/CT imaging in 30 patients with various cancers, we concluded that the image quality with 8 min acquisition can meet the diagnostic requirements. To further verify the rationality and operability of this conclusion, a group of patients with colorectal cancer with TB PET/CT imaging using the conventional activity was selected as the reference. A comparative study was conducted on the image information and lesion detection efficiency of patients who underwent 1/10 activity of TB PET/CT imaging, to verify the feasibility of 8 min acquisition in clinical application.

Eleven patients with colorectal cancer underwent 1/10 activity of ^{18}F-FDG TB PET/CT imaging, including seven men and four women, who had a mean BMI of 22.75 ± 3.46 kg/m^2, an average of fasting blood glucose level of 5.81 ± 0.61 mmol/L, a mean injection activity of 24.79 ± 4.44 MBq, and the mean uptake time post injection was 62.91 ± 5.50 min. All patients were pathologically confirmed to be suffering from colorectal cancer, including 10 cases of medium to highly differentiated adenocarcinoma and 1 case of high-grade intraepithelial neoplasia.

In the matched study, 11 patients with colorectal cancer who received TB PET/CT imaging at routine activity (3.7 MBq/kg) ^{18}F-FDG were selected from the database, and matched with the same demographics such as sex, height, weight, BMI, blood glucose, waiting time after injection of the imaging agent, tumor pathological type, and the degree of differentiation of the 11 patients with colorectal cancer in the 1/10 activity group. The seven men and four women in the routine activity group included 10 cases of medium to highly differentiated adenocarcinoma and 1 case of high-grade intraepithelial neoplasia. Their mean BMI was 25.00 ± 3.92 kg/m^2, the average of fasting blood glucose level was 5.31 ± 0.53 mmol/L, the mean injection activity was 271.21 ± 61.42 MBq, and the mean uptake time post injection was 58.00 ± 5.57 min. To reduce the comparison bias, the following exclusion criteria were strictly followed for case selection: No uptake of FDG in primary lesions, disease in the liver precluding measurement of quantitative metrics in the normal liver, BMI ≥30 kg/m^2, blood glucose level >7.0 mmol/L, and an FDG uptake time of more than 70 min. All information was matched between the 1/10 activity group and the routine activity group except for the difference in injection activity.

Our previous research reported that the routine activity TB PET images with 2 min acquisition could meet the needs of clinical diagnosis [8]. Therefore, PET images acquired within 2 min in the routine activity group and the PET images acquired within 8 min in the 1/10 activity group were compared and analyzed in this study.

The PET image quality was evaluated subjectively and PET parameters were measured, respectively. The subjective scoring criteria and parameter measurement methods were the same as in Sect. 7.1.

The results of subjective evaluation by the two raters showed that the image quality of 1/10 activity TB PET/CT imaging at 8 min was not inferior to that of the routine activity at 2 min. The image quality scores of the 1/10 activity group at 8 min and the routine activity group at 2 min were 3.91 ± 0.30 and 3.82 ± 0.60, respectively. The subjective scores were comparable between the two groups (P = 0.311). The analysis of objective parameters demonstrated that the lesion SUV_{max} and TBR values of the 1/10 activity group were 23.43 ± 8.64 and 7.07 ± 2.74, respectively, and those of the routine activity group were 24.22 ± 12.15 and 7.56 ± 3.51, respectively. No significant difference was found between the two groups. Liver SUV_{mean} and SD values in the 1/10 activity group were 2.78 ± 0.33 and 0.21 ± 0.05, and in the routine activity group, they were 2.84 ± 0.47 and 0.23 ± 0.08, respectively. The results of two groups were comparable (P = 0.747 and 0.544, respectively). The SNR values of the 1/10 activity group and routine activity group were 13.77 ± 2.14 and 13.40 ± 2.90, respectively. There was no statistical difference between the two groups (P = 0.716).

It was further confirmed that the image quality of 1/10 activity TB PET/CT acquisition at 8 min was equivalent to that of the routine activity acquisition at 2 min by clinical validation analysis (Fig. 7.2). The results of lesion display and the semi-quantitative analysis were generally consistent, indicating that 1/10 activity of ^{18}F-FDG TB PET/CT acquisition at 8 min could be the optional imaging conditions.

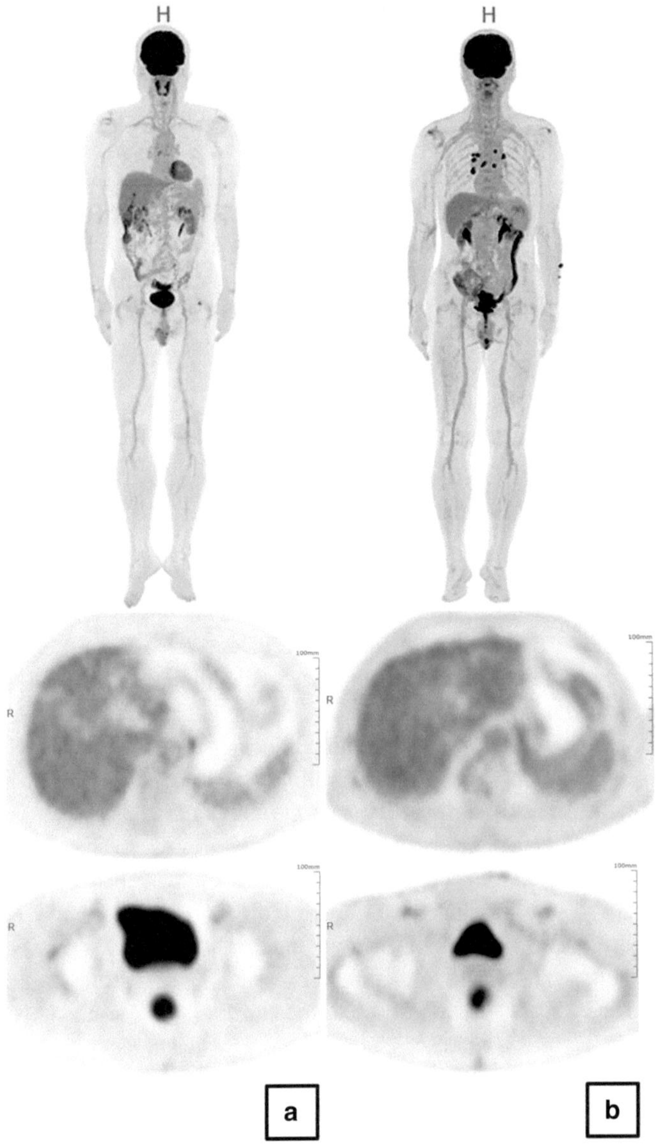

Fig. 7.2 Comparison between 1/10 activity TB PET/CT images and routine full activity TB PET/CT images. (**a**) PET images of a 56-year-old man with rectal adenocarcinoma (grade II–III). Whole-body coronal maximum intensity projection (MIP) of PET, transverse view of the liver, and transverse view of the lesion which was acquired for 8 min with 1/10 activity. (**b**) PET images of a 54-year-old man with rectal adenocarcinoma (grade II–III). PET images of whole-body coronal MIP, transverse view of the liver, and transverse view of the lesion acquired for 2 min with routine fulle activity. The results show that the image quality of 1/10 activity scanned for 8 min was comparable to that of the full activity scanned for 2 min

7.3 Clinical Application of TB PET/CT Imaging with 1/10 Activity ^{18}F-FDG

The 1/10 activity TB PET/CT imaging could be clinically applied to radiation-sensitive populations such as infants, children, adolescents, and those who need multiple PET/CT examinations in a short period of time.

7.3.1 The Application of 1/10 Activity of ^{18}F-FDG TB PET/CT Imaging in Children

Growth and development are distinct physiological phenomena in children, whose disease spectrum and biological characteristics are significantly different from those of adults. Tumors in adults often originate from epithelial tissue, while tumors in children are mostly embryonic and are more common in the hematological system, central nervous system, and sympathetic nervous system. Neuroblastoma, which originates in the post-ganglionic sympathetic nervous system, is one of the most common extracranial solid malignancies in pediatric patients, with incidences ranked in first and second place in infants younger than 1 year old and in children ages 1–4 years old, respectively [9]. Neuroblastoma is characterized by high heterogeneity, high malignancy, and rapid progression. It has mostly advanced to the middle or late stages at diagnosis and approximately 10% of primary lesions are undetectable. Diagnosis, treatment, and prognosis of neuroblastoma are affected by many factors, including tumor size, primary location, degree of spread, and genetic variation. Following the principle of multidisciplinary therapeutics, comprehensive treatment protocols are employed currently in clinical practice, including surgery, chemotherapy, radiotherapy, hematopoietic stem cell transplantation, and immunotherapy. PET/CT plays a key role in finding primary tumor lesions, staging, efficacy evaluation, and long-term follow-up (Fig. 7.3), and particularly to distinguish residual tumor tissue from scars after surgery, which is better than conventional magnetic resonance imaging (MRI) and CT. In addition, TB PET/CT imaging has the advantage of greatly reducing the radiation dose to children using only 1/10 activity of the ^{18}F-FDG.

^{18}F-FDG is a radiolabeled analog of glucose, and as a nonspecific tracer, it can be used not only for tumor imaging, but also for the diagnosis and evaluation of benign diseases, such as inflammation or infection. Fever is one of the most common symptoms seen in children, mainly resulting from infectious diseases in children under the age of 6. The proportion of non-infectious inflammatory conditions increases with age and becomes the main cause of Fever of Undetermined Origin (FUO) in children over 6 years of age. Previous studies showed that 25–91% of children with FUO might obtain a final diagnosis using ^{18}F-FDG PET/CT imaging [10]. The wide range of the percentages may also suggest that FDG-PET has greater application and room for improvement in the diagnosis of FUO in children. Takayasu arteritis is a chronic, progressive, and nonspecific inflammation mainly involving the aorta and its branches, which manifests as active inflammation in the early stage, and gradually causes narrowing, occlusion, and dilation of blood vessels over time. Clinical symptoms in children are mostly fever, hypertension, and weight loss; however, clinical manifestations and signs are often atypical. The American College of Rheumatology (ACR) classification standards are more applicable to adults, while in pediatric clinical practice, the European League Against Rheumatism (EULAR)-Pediatric Rheumatology European Society (PReS)-Pediatric Rheumatology International Trials Organization (PRINTO) classification standard developed at the 2008 Ankara meeting is used more often. Takayasu arteritis is classified into four clinical types, based on the location and extent of the arteritis: Type I, involving in aortic arch and its three main branches; Type II, involving in thoracic-abdominal aorta; Type III, with extensive aortic involvement; and Type IV, involving in the pulmonary artery. However, the existing diagnostic and classification criteria have certain limitations, which brings difficulties to clinical practice. Early diagnosis and early treatment is vital [11]. In PET imaging, there is no obvious ^{18}F-FDG uptake in the normal vascular wall, but when an inflammatory response occurs, the activity at the lesion site of the vascular wall will increase (Fig. 7.4). The diagnosis of this disease is often elusive; therefore, TB PET/CT imaging is particularly valuable for the diagnosis of atypical cases. 1/10 activity FDG TB PET/CT imaging and delayed imaging have significant advantages in the diagnosis and evaluation of Takayasu arteritis in children.

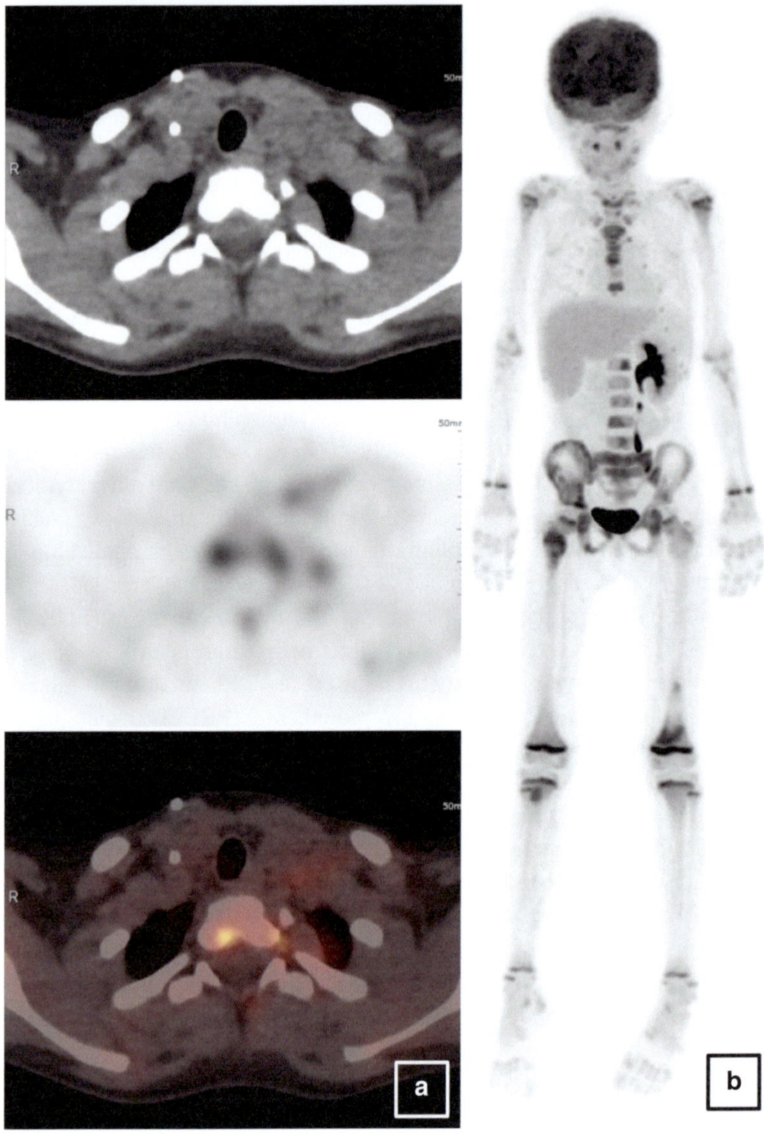

Fig. 7.3 TB PET/CT imaging with 1/10 activity in children with neuroblastoma. A 7-year-old boy underwent radical resection of right retroperitoneal neuroblastoma 3 years ago in another hospital, followed by several courses of postoperative chemotherapy and radiotherapy in the surgical area. PET/CT was performed for re-staging. His body weight was 17.6 kg and the injection activity of ^{18}F-FDG was 6.8 MBq. The PET/CT results indicated metastasis in left cervical lymph node with an SUV_{max} of 2.6 (**a**); multiple bone metastases were observed in the spine, pelvic bones, and the bones of the four limbs (**b**)

7.3.2 The Application of 1/10 Activity of ^{18}F-FDG TB PET/CT Imaging in the Therapeutic Evaluation of Lymphoma

Lymphoma is a malignant tumor originating from the lymphatic system and is the most common malignant tumor of the hematological system. It usually occurs in lymph nodes, but also in tissues or organs outside lymph nodes, such as the stomach, intestine, lung, brain, bone, and skin. The main clinical manifestation is painless and progressive lymphadenopathy, which might be accompanied by low fever, night sweats, emaciation, and other symptoms. The 2016 World Health Organization (WHO) classification of lymphoma histiocytic tumors divides it into precursor lymphocytic tumors (B lymphoblastic leukemia/lymphoma and T lymphoblastic leukemia/lymphoma), mature B cell tumors, mature T and natural killer (NK) cell malignant tumors, Hodgkin's lymphoma, post-transplantation lymphoproliferative disorder, and histiocytic and dendritic cell malignant tumors.

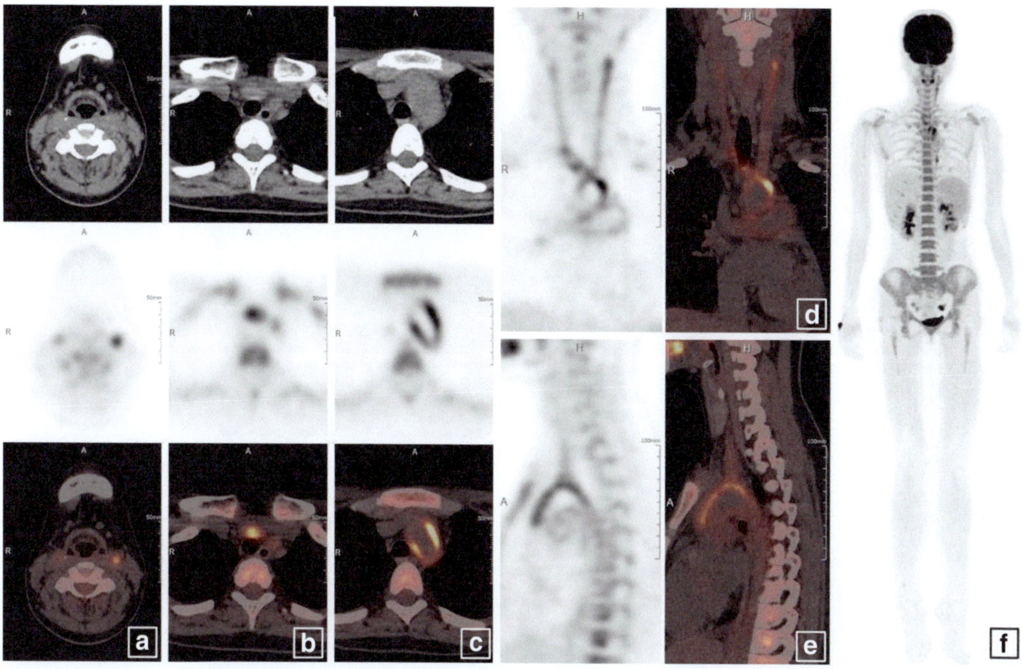

Fig. 7.4 TB ^{18}F-FDG PET/CT image acquired with 1/10 activity in a child with multiple Takayasu arteritis. A 15-year-old girl with a 2-month history of fever underwent 1/10-activity TB ^{18}F-FDG PET/CT imaging to determine the etiology. Her body weight was 54.0 kg and the injected activity of ^{18}F-FDG was 20.1 MBq. PET/CT images show increased ^{18}F-FDG uptake in the thickened local walls of the bilateral common carotid artery, the brachiocephalic trunk, and the aortic arch, with the SUV_{max} reached 8.5 (**a**–**f**). Combined with age, abnormal pulse, blood pressure discrepancy between her upper limbs, vascular bruits, and the elevated acute-phase inflammatory reactants, multiple Takayasu arteritis was clinically diagnosed according to the EULAR-PReS-PRINTO criteria

Lymphoma has high heterogeneity; therefore, different types of lymphoma have different treatment options. The main treatments for lymphoma include chemotherapy, radiotherapy, bone marrow transplantation, and surgery. Currently, the most commonly used treatment is combined chemotherapy. PET/CT imaging was used to evaluate the efficacy of lymphoma diagnosis and treatment in the 2007 version of lymphoma diagnosis and treatment evaluation criteria. Subsequently, the Deauville 5-PS criteria for invasive lymphoma with abnormal increased glucose metabolism was proposed in 2009, and in 2014, the Lugano criteria were proposed to evaluate the efficacy of lymphoma, including aggressive lymphoma, indolent lymphoma, and some lymphoma with no uptake of imaging agents [12, 13].

The efficacy evaluation of lymphoma using PET/CT includes three stages: baseline evaluation, mid-term evaluation, and post-treatment efficacy evaluation. It is recommended to perform baseline evaluation before treatment for lymphoma with significant ^{18}F-FDG uptake. It is not only used for lymphoma staging and guiding the clinic to draw up a rational treatment regimen, but also provides a baseline for the subsequent mid-term evaluation and post-treatment evaluation (Fig. 7.5). The mid-term evaluation can assess the effectiveness of chemotherapy regimens and guide subsequent treatment decisions. The NCCN guidelines recommend that two or four cycles of ABVD regimen (doxorubicin hydrochloride (Adriamycin), bleomycin sulfate, vinblastine sulfate, and dacarbazine) or four cycles of the enhanced BEACOPP regimen (bleomycin sulfate, etoposide phosphate, doxorubicin hydrochloride (Adriamycin), cyclophosphamide, vincristine sulfate (Oncovin), procarbazine hydrochloride,

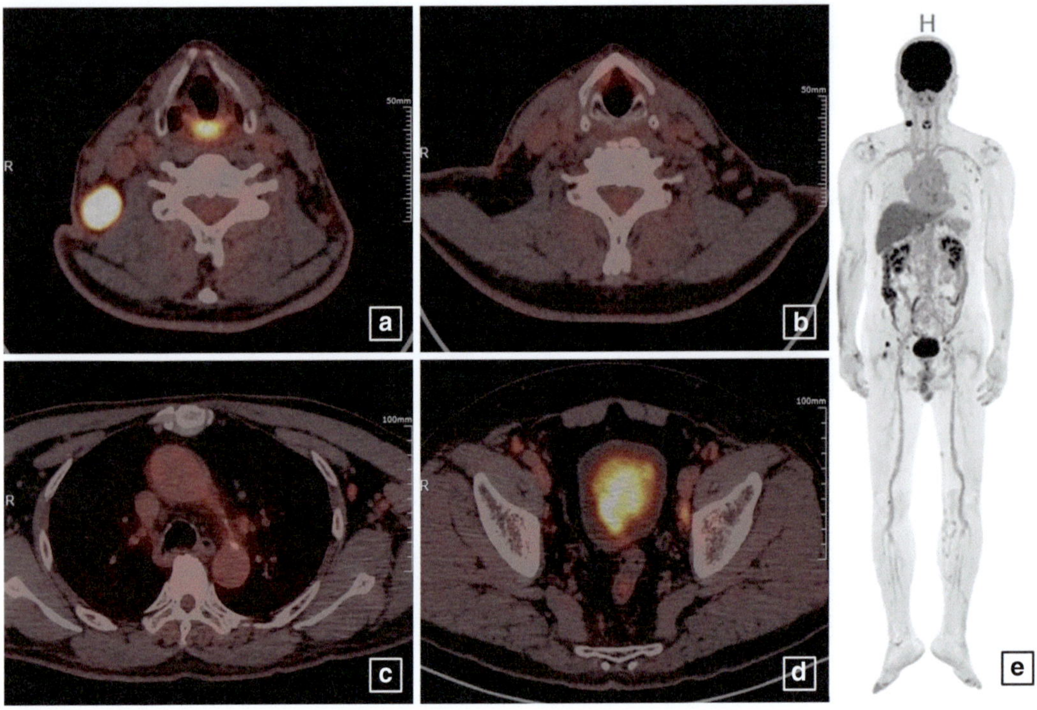

Fig. 7.5 Baseline examination for lymphoma performed using 1/10 activity TB PET/CT. A 73-year-old man whose chief complaint was a neck mass for more than 1 month underwent PET/CT imaging to assist diagnosis. The patient's weight was 67 kg and the injected ^{18}F-FDG activity was 25.8 MBq. PET/CT images showed lymphoma involving the lymph node in the right posterior cervical triangle, with an SUV_{max} of 12.8 (**a**). Bilateral cervical, axillary, and pelvic lymph nodes might be involved with the SUV_{max} being 4.9 (**b–e**). Subsequently, the right cervical lymph node was resected and pathologically confirmed as diffuse large B cell lymphoma

and prednisone) should be followed by PET/CT imaging for mid-term evaluation [14], and the treatment regimen was adjusted according to the Deauville score (Fig. 7.6). PET/CT can effectively distinguish between residual or recurrent tumors and residual scar tissue after treatment and provide the basis for subsequent treatment (Fig. 7.7).

Lymphoma patients usually need to undergo multiple PET/CT imaging at different time points from diagnosis, staging, re-staging to efficacy evaluation, which will undoubtedly increase the radiation dose to the patients. The 1/10 activity TB PET/CT greatly reduces the radiation dose caused by PET tracers, thus its application provides good news for these patients, especially pediatric patients.

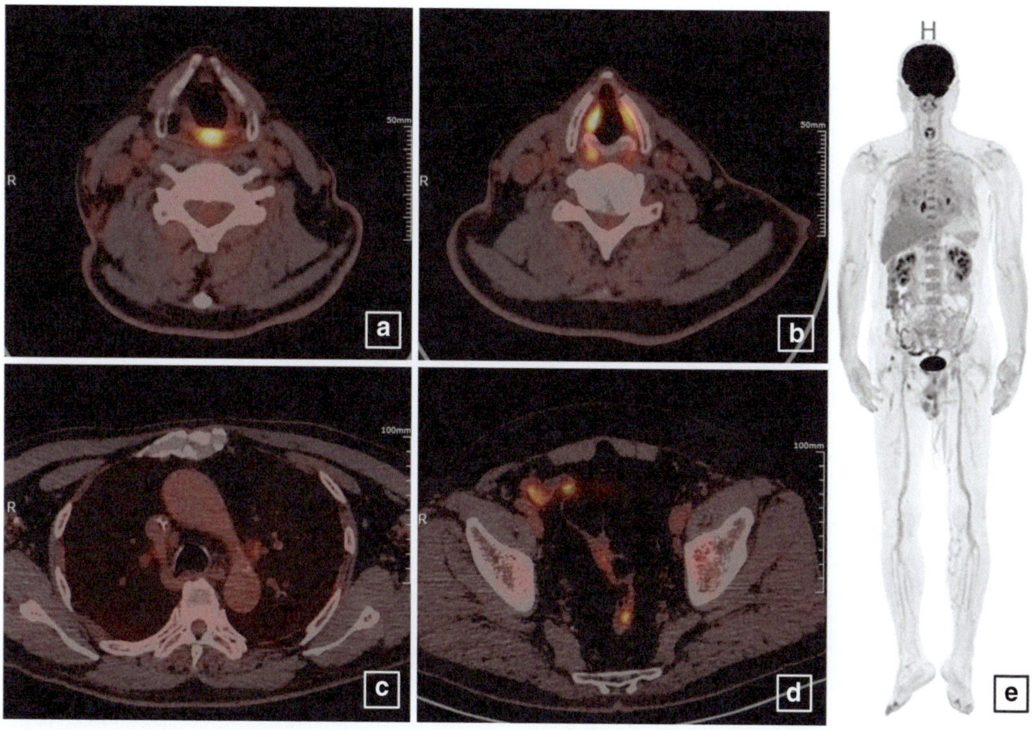

Fig. 7.6 Mid-term therapy assessment of patient with lymphoma using 1/10 activity TB PET/CT. The case from Fig. 7.5 underwent PET/CT examination again after three cycles of chemotherapy. The original pathological lymph node in the right posterior cervical triangle was dissected by surgery (**a**). The remaining lymph nodes in bilateral neck, in the clavicular region, in the axillary fossa, and in the pelvis reduced with smaller sizes than before, in addition with reduced glucose metabolism, with the maximum SUV_{max} of all lesions being 2.0 (**b–e**)

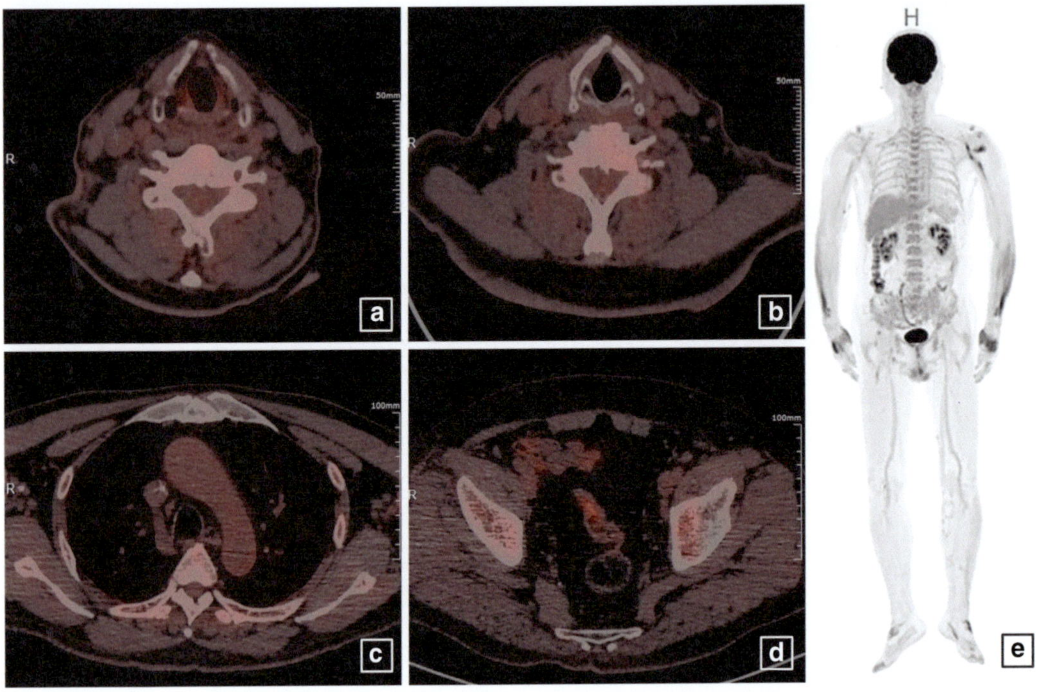

Fig. 7.7 Therapy evaluation using 1/10-activity TB PET/CT for a patient with lymphoma. The case from Fig. 7.6 underwent PET/CT examination after additional two cycles of chemotherapy. The original lymph node in the right posterior cervical triangle was dissected by surgery (**a**). The remaining lymph nodes in bilateral neck, in the clavicular region, and in the axillary fossa almost disappeared (**b, c**), while the lymph nodes in the pelvis were similar to those before, with the maximum SUV_{max} of all lesions being 1.6 (**d–e**)

References

1. Karakatsanis NA, Fokou E, Tsoumpas C. Dosage optimization in positron emission tomography: state-of-the-art methods and future prospects. Am J Nucl Med Mol Imaging. 2015;5(5):527–47.
2. Huang B, Law MW, Khong P. Whole-body PET/CT scanning: estimation of radiation dose and cancer risk. Radiology. 2009;251(1):166–74.
3. Alessio AM, Sammer M, Phillips GS, Manchanda V, Mohr BC, Parisi MT. Evaluation of optimal acquisition duration or injected activity for pediatric ^{18}F-FDG PET/CT. J Nucl Med. 2011;52(7):1028–34.
4. Spencer BA, Berg E, Schmall JP, Omidvari N, Leung EK, Abdelhafez YG, et al. Performance evaluation of the uEXPLORER total-body PET/CT scanner based on NEMA NU 2-2018 with additional tests to characterize PET scanners with a long axial field of view. J Nucl Med. 2021;62(6):861–70.
5. Badawi RD, Shi H, Hu P, Chen S, Xu T, Price PM, et al. First human imaging studies with the EXPLORER total-body PET scanner. J Nucl Med. 2019;60(3):299–303.
6. Zhang X, Zhou J, Cherry SR, Badawi RD, Qi J. Quantitative image reconstruction for total-body PET imaging using the 2-meter long EXPLORER scanner. Phys Med Biol. 2017;62(6):2465–85.
7. Hu Y, Liu G, Yu H, Wang Y, Li C, Tan H, et al. Feasibility of acquisitions using total-body PET/CT with an ultra-low ^{18}F-FDG activity. J Nucl Med. 2022;63(6):959–65.
8. Zhang Y, Hu P, Wu R, Gu Y, Chen S, Yu H, et al. The image quality, lesion detectability, and acquisition time of ^{18}F-FDG total-body PET/CT in oncological patients. Eur J Nucl Med Mol Imaging. 2020;47(11):2507–15.
9. Ni X, Li Z, Li X, Zhang X, Bai G, Liu Y, et al. Socioeconomic inequalities in cancer incidence and access to health services among children and adolescents in China: a cross-sectional study. Lancet. 2022;400(10357):1020–32.
10. Houseni M, Chamroonrat W, Servaes S, Alavi A, Zhuang H. Applications of PET/CT in pediatric patients with fever of unknown origin. Pet Clin. 2008;3(4):605–19.
11. Zucker EJ, Chan FP. Pediatric cardiothoracic vasculitis: multimodality imaging review. Pediatr Radiol. 2022;52(10):1895–909.

12. Cheson BD, Fisher RI, Barrington SF, Cavalli F, Schwartz LH, Zucca E, et al. Recommendations for initial evaluation, staging, and response assessment of Hodgkin and non-Hodgkin lymphoma: the Lugano classification. J Clin Oncol. 2014;32(27):3059–68.
13. Juweid ME, Wiseman GA, Vose JM, Ritchie JM, Menda Y, Wooldridge JE, et al. Response assessment of aggressive non-Hodgkin's lymphoma by integrated International Workshop Criteria and fluorine-18-fluorodeoxyglucose positron emission tomography. J Clin Oncol. 2005;23(21):4652–61.
14. Hoppe RT, Advani RH, Ai WZ, Ambinder RF, Armand P, Bello CM, et al. Hodgkin lymphoma, version 2.2020, NCCN clinical practice guidelines in oncology. J Natl Compr Cancer Netw. 2020;18(6):755–81.

8 Exploration of Application Technology in Total-Body PET/CT

Shuguang Chen, Guobing Liu, Haojun Yu, Chi Qi, Xiuli Sui, and Yan Hu

In comparison to traditional positron emission tomography–computed tomography (PET/CT), total-body (TB) PET/CT has demonstrated higher sensitivity and offers a variety of imaging parameters, such as ultra-low dose scanning, fast scanning, and ultra-long time-delay scanning. This expansion of PET/CT's clinical application is noteworthy; however, further exploration and improvement of TB PET/CT are necessary to maximize its capabilities.

8.1 Application of a Gating Approach in TB PET/CT Imaging

The finite axial field of view (AFOV) and limited sensitivity of traditional PET imaging can lead to extended scan times and the inability to achieve breath-hold acquisition with standard injection doses. Respiratory motion during PET image acquisition can cause adjacent organs or lesions near the diaphragm and chest wall to become blurred, thus diminishing image quality [1]. Furthermore, the temporal disparity between CT and PET acquisition of images of the same tissue or organ, combined with the effects of respiratory motion, can lead to discrepancies in their location and shape, thereby compromising registration accuracy. Additionally, the use of poorly registered CT images for attenuation correction (AC) of PET images can result in bias and quantitative inaccuracies.

The implementation of respiratory gating technology has been demonstrated to be effective in reducing image artifacts caused by respiratory motion. Hardware-assisted gating, which involves the utilization of external devices, such as an elastic band with a pressure sensor placed on the patient's chest or abdomen to detect changes in pressure signals during inhalation and exhalation, has been shown to yield benefits including increased lesion standardized uptake values (SUVs), reduced metabolic tumor volume (MTV), decreased image noise, and improved diagnostic efficacy compared with nongated acquisition. However, the complexity of the external devices, the time-consuming nature of the process, and the inconsistency of the movement of organs in the thoracic and abdominal cavities, as well as the narrow effective time window collected in each respiratory cycle, can lead to a lower PET image signal-to-noise ratio (SNR) and increased image acquisition time. In recent years, data-driven gating (DDG) has been proposed as an alternative to hardware-assisted gating [2]. This technique is based on the temporal and spatial distribution characteristics of PET counts, which are used to extract effective "respiratory waveforms" and retain those counts with relatively small motion amplitude during the

S. Chen · G. Liu (✉) · H. Yu · C. Qi · X. Sui · Y. Hu
Department of Nuclear Medicine, Zhongshan Hospital, Fudan University, Shanghai, China
e-mail: liu.guobing@zs-hospital.sh.cn

© Shanghai Scientific and Technical Publishers 2024
H. Shi et al. (eds.), *Total-Body PET/CT*, https://doi.org/10.1007/978-981-97-5065-8_8

"respiratory cycle" for PET image reconstruction. The advantage of DDG is that it does not require any additional hardware and does not increase the workload of PET imaging workflow, making it easier in clinical application. However, DDG requires sufficient counts to ensure that the PET image reconstruction needs are met. For traditional PET/CT devices, this necessitates a longer PET acquisition time (about 3–4 times) for the lower chest and upper abdomen, which is difficult to promote in clinical application. Conversely, TB PET/CT has the significant advantage of providing sufficient counts for DDG reconstruction even under conventional acquisition time. Furthermore, if the acquisition time is appropriately prolonged (single-bed with total-body coverage) to ensure the quality of the DDG reconstructed image, the total scan time will not be significantly increased. Therefore, the application of DDG respiratory gating technology in TB PET/CT imaging is a promising investigatory technique; however, its precise value requires further research and exploration.

TB PET/CT significantly improves detector sensitivity and PET image quality, and the significant improvement in count detection efficiency has created conditions conducive to the application of respiratory gating imaging techniques.

8.1.1 The Application of Respiratory Gating in TB PET/CT Imaging of Chest and Abdominal Tumors

Respiratory motion during PET/CT examinations of the chest and abdomen can cause the diaphragm to oscillate by 8–25 mm, leading to respiratory motion artifacts that detrimentally affect the image quality of organs in the upper abdomen and lower chest, potentially obscuring small lesions. The implementation of respiratory gating technology in clinical settings can mitigate these issues and significantly enhance PET image quality.

The emergence of TB PET/CT technology and the enhancement of its capabilities have enabled the use of respiratory gating techniques to acquire high-quality images for clinical applications. This approach surpasses traditional respiratory gating devices, which rely on an external device to extract respiratory waveforms and select the end-expiration phase as a relatively static phase to acquire PET images with minimal displacement. The traditional method has certain drawbacks, such as a limited acquisition window that might not provide adequate counts and necessitate longer PET acquisition times, as well as the need for high-frequency uniformity, which can be difficult for patients with underlying respiratory diseases.

Respiratory gating can be used to divide the respiratory waveform obtained from an external device into three distinct time windows, as shown in Fig. 8.1, with the second time window corresponding to the end-expiratory phase and triggering PET image acquisition. The acquired time window is equivalent to one-third of the nongated acquisition time. At our center, we investigated the application value of gated TB PET/CT acquisition for the diagnosis of abdominal tumors. After analyzing the lesion detection rate, semi-quantitative analysis, and image quality, we discovered that 15-min gated PET acquisition yielded superior image quality compared with 15-min nongated PET acquisition. Furthermore, 6-min gated PET acquisition was found to produce a lesion detection rate and image quality comparable to that of 15-min gated PET imaging (Fig. 8.2).

In conclusion, the application of respiratory-gated ^{18}F-FDG TB PET/CT imaging is a viable and practical technique that significantly improves PET image quality, thereby indicating its potential for clinical application.

8.1.2 Application of Dual-Gated Technology in TB PET/CT Cardiac Imaging

Compared with single-photon emission computed tomography (SPECT), PET offers higher sensitivity, and spatial and temporal resolution, and thus is a promising tool for diagnosing and evaluating cardiovascular diseases. However, the

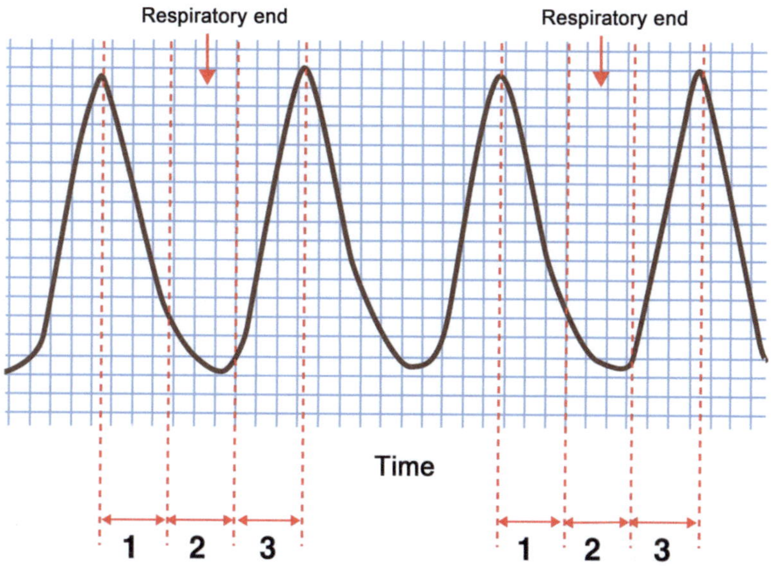

Fig. 8.1 Schematic diagram of time windows for respiratory gating acquisition

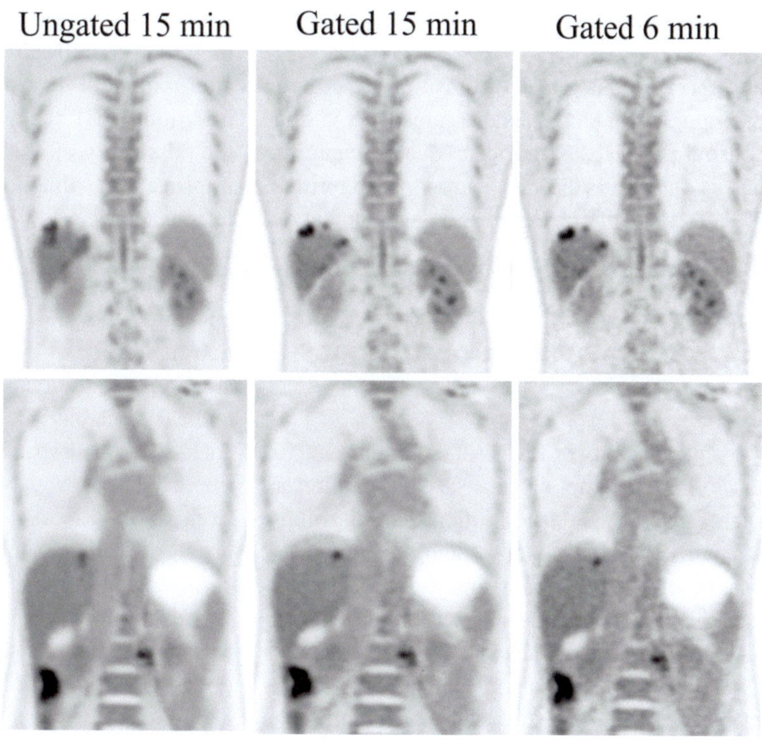

Fig. 8.2 Comparison of TB PET/CT imaging for malignant abdominal tumors under different acquisition conditions

physiological contraction of the heart and respiratory motion present challenges in obtaining high-quality PET images, necessitating longer acquisition times. During PET/CT imaging, attenuation correction of PET images can be improved with the aid of CT; however, since CT and PET images are not acquired simultaneously, registration errors might occur because of disparities in morphology and position between the two modalities.

The application of dual-gated technology, incorporating electrocardiogram and/or respiratory gating, is deemed the ideal way to minimize motion artifacts. Nevertheless, it significantly increases the time required to acquire adequate counts, thereby placing higher demands on imaging equipment. Recently, motion correction methods based on TB PET/CT imaging have been proposed, which can effectively amalgamate both respiratory gating and electrocardiogram gating to achieve an ideal balance between motion correction and image quality. TB PET/CT electrocardiogram gating uses a three-lead electrocardiogram for gated reconstruction.

The dual-gate control technology in the TB PET/CT imaging system has the potential to minimize the deleterious effects of motion on image quality. During the image reconstruction process, the raw data is typically divided into 16–64 data blocks, the exact number of which is contingent upon the number of respiratory and cardiac gates used.

However, dual-gated acquisition is still an emerging technology and is subject to various constraints, such as the technique of capturing gated data and the reconstruction algorithm. Therefore, further research and development are warranted in this field.

8.2 Small-Voxel Reconstruction of TB PET Images

The image quality of PET is of paramount importance for accurate diagnosis, with parameters such as SNR, spatial resolution, partial volume effect (PVE), and target-to-non-target ratio (T/NT) being used for evaluation. In clinical applications, the imaging matrix used can have a considerable impact on image quality. Therefore, it is essential to strike a balance between the abovementioned parameters to achieve optimal image quality. The limited AFOV of conventional PET and its associated physical and technical characteristics result in inherently low spatial resolution and photon detection efficiency, making it difficult to detect small lesions using large imaging matrices. However, with the continual advancement of technology, improved hardware and software with enhanced performance can be applied to improve image quality, such as PET scanners with longer AFOV; more scintillation crystals and photomultiplier tubes with higher detection efficiency; the application of time-of-flight (TOF) [3] and point spread function (PSF) analysis [4], and new reconstruction algorithms [5, 6].

Conventional PET scanners, with an AFOV ranging from 15 to 30 cm, have been found to have limited coverage and a relatively low photon detection efficiency [7]. Despite this, several studies have evaluated the potential of using small voxels, such as $2 \times 2 \times 2$ mm^3 in conventional PET/CT to improve the accuracy of small lesion detection [8, 9]. TB PET/CT, with its 194 cm AFOV has significantly increased the effective counting rate, which is approximately 40 times higher than that of a traditional PET scanner [10, 11]. This provides the possibility of using small-voxel imaging to improve the diagnostic accuracy of small lesions (Fig. 8.3).

Our center conducted an exploratory study to assess the feasibility of using $1.2 \times 1.2 \times 1.4$ mm^3 and $0.6 \times 0.6 \times 1.4$ mm^3 small-voxel reconstruction for TB PET/CT imaging, optimizing reconstruction conditions through modeling and clinical research. The results of the study indicated that small-voxel TB PET/CT imaging can improve the SUV_{max} of lesions and the tumor-to-liver ratio (TLR) and is advantageous for diagnosing small or low-metabolism lesions if sufficient counts are acquired. Furthermore, it was determined that for ^{18}F-fluorodeoxyglucose (FDG) injections at the recommended standard dose (3.7 MBq/kg), a 5-min acquisition time with a voxel size of $1.2 \times 1.2 \times 1.4$ mm^3 for image reconstruction or an 8-min acquisition time with a voxel size of $0.6 \times 0.6 \times 1.4$ mm^3 for image reconstruction can yield images that meet clinical diagnostic requirements.

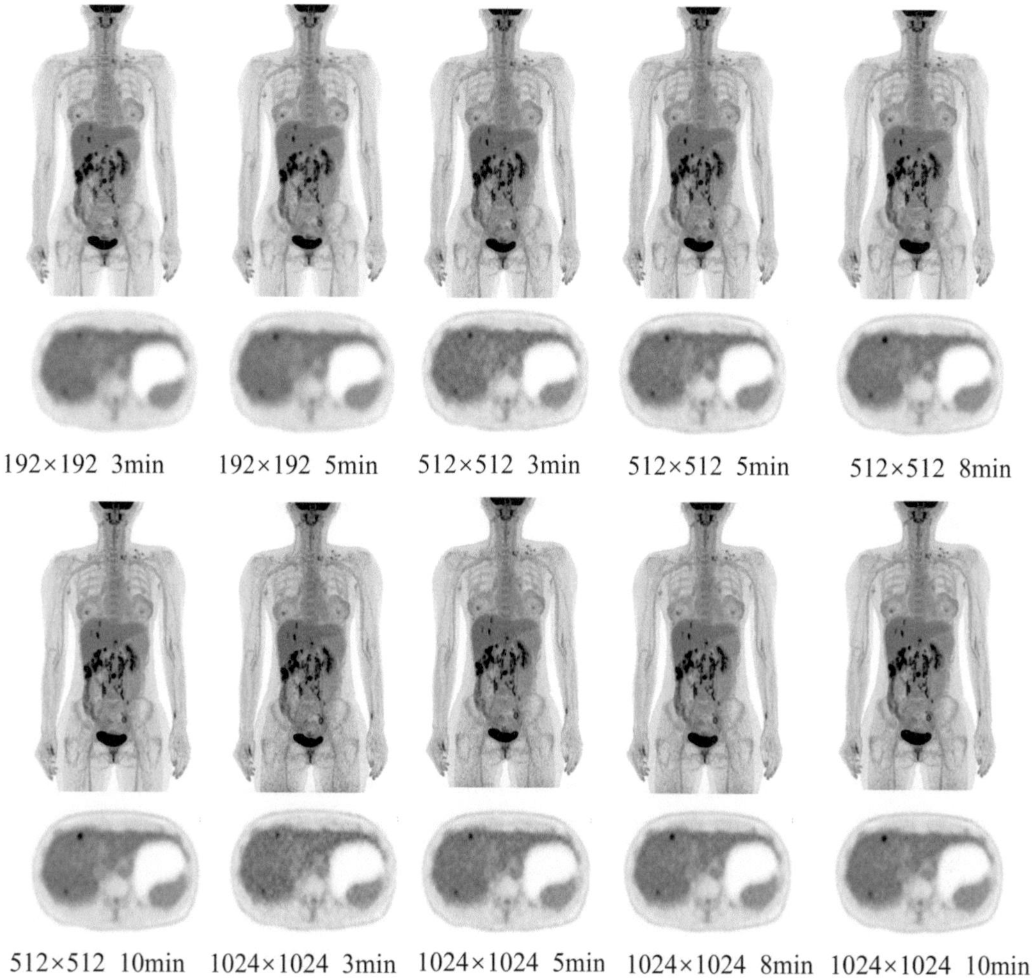

Fig. 8.3 Small-voxel reconstruction improves contrast and image SNR for visualization of liver lesion. A 28-year-old female patient with pathologically confirmed moderately-to-poorly differentiated colon adenocarcinoma underwent a PET/CT scan for staging

8.3 Optimization of TB PET Imaging Reconstruction Parameters with Ultra-Low (1/10) Dose

The clinical application of long AFOV PET has enabled imaging at 1/10th of the recommended dose (3.7 MBq/kg) to become a viable option in practice. A critical question in clinical practice is how to construct appropriate reconstruction parameters for ultra-low dose imaging to achieve the highest image quality.

A subject with a height of 152 cm and a weight of 43.5 kg was injected with 25 MBq (0.57 MBq/kg) of ^{18}F-FDG and underwent a 10-min uEXPLORER TB PET imaging, as reported in the literature [12]. Ordered Subset Expectation Maximization (OSEM) is the most commonly used image reconstruction technique in PET clinical practice. OSEM is characterized by an increase in noise with the number of iterations when the count rate is relatively low. If only one or two iterations are performed, the contrast recovery is insufficient and the lesion cannot be adequately visualized [13, 14]. Therefore, a balance must be struck between image noise and quantitative accuracy, which often leads to insufficient image convergence.

Our previous clinical practice demonstrated that TB PET/CT imaging with an ultra-low dose (0.37 MBq/kg) for 15 min and reconstruction using the OSEM algorithm can yield high-quality images [15]. However, as the subject's weight increased, the noise-equivalent count rate (NECR) decreased rapidly [16]. Reconstructions for patients with a larger body mass index (BMI) consistently resulted in poor image quality when using the OSEM algorithm, thus making it inadequate for clinical diagnosis [17]. To address this deficiency, a new Bayesian penalized likelihood reconstruction algorithm (HYPER Iterative) was proposed [18]. This algorithm incorporates noise control into each iteration and finds the maximum likelihood solution through repeated iterations, thereby significantly suppressing noise while achieving optimal convergence.

A cohort of ultra-low dose (0.37 MBq/kg) ^{18}F-FDG TB PET/CT images were subjected to an analysis of image quality and lesion detectability by our team, with different reconstructions being employed. The results showed that OSEM reconstructions with three iterations were sufficient to meet the clinical criteria for patients with a BMI <29.9. For those with a BMI $\geq$30, it is recommended that the HYPER Iteration algorithm (with a β-value ranging from 0.3 to 0.5) be used to ensure consistent visual image quality and quantitative assessment.

8.4 Application of Low-Dose CT in TB PET/CT Imaging

As the clinical application of PET/CT continues to expand, the radiation dose has become a matter of concern, particularly for radiation-sensitive populations, such as children and adolescents, and those undergoing multiple PET/CT examinations for evaluation and treatment. The radiation dose from PET/CT is derived from the X-rays emitted during the CT scan and the gamma rays produced by the PET imaging agent, with the radiation dose from the CT scan constituting the majority [19]. Strategies to reduce the radiation dose from the CT scan include tube current modulation, tube voltage reduction, pitch increment and noise reduction filters, and new reconstruction algorithms [20, 21].

Previous reports have indicated that despite the diagnostic information yielded by images being largely consistent regardless of the tube current used, a decrease in the tube current will result in an increase in image noise and a decrease in image quality [22, 23]. Moreover, the implementation of tube current automatic modulation technology was observed to have an effect on the radiation dose along the Z-axis, depending on the direction of the localizing image. It was observed that when the arms are placed on the top of the head, the radiation dose is reduced.

In addition, reducing the tube voltage can also lead to a decrease in radiation dose; however, this will also result in a decrease in image contrast and uniformity. To counter this, an adaptive statistical iterative reconstruction algorithm, such as hybrid iterative reconstruction (HIR), can be employed to reduce the radiation dose while still maintaining a high level of image clarity and diagnostic accuracy. HIR works by optimizing raw data in the projection domains through iteration loops, which include a scanner model, a statistical noise model, and projection noise estimation [24].

The Artificial Intelligence Iterative Reconstruction (AIIR) algorithm, a deep-learning-based reconstruction algorithm, was initially developed to produce images with reduced noise and enhanced low contrast detectability via the use of both standards and stimulated multi-dose level CT images. In comparison with conventional dose CT images, the AIIR algorithm is capable of denoising low-dose images while maintaining image quality. Therefore, our center preliminarily explored the application of the AIIR algorithm in low-dose CT image reconstruction in clinical practice, involving PET/CT images from 52 patients (23 females with an average age of 21–86 years; 29 males with an average age of 41–86 years). All examinations were performed on the TB PET/CT scanner, uEXPLORER (United Imaging Healthcare), equipped with 80 rows and a 128-slice CT. The patient lay in the supine position and underwent a CT scout scan to correct the positioning, followed by an attenuation correction CT scan for PET attenuation correction. The PET images were acquired over 10 min. Subsequently, the range of standard-dose CT for the anatomical location was scanned from the top of the skull to the middle femur. The scanning protocol of the total-body ultra-low-dose CT was set as a tube voltage of 120 kV, a tube current of 10 mA, a gantry rotation time of 0.5 s, a beam pitch of 1.0125, a slice thickness of 1.0 mm, and a field of view (FOV) of 500 mm. The acquisition protocol of standard-dose CT was a tube voltage of 120 kV, auto modulation tube current technology, a gantry rotation time of 0.5 s, a beam pitch of 0.9875, a slice thickness of 1.0 mm, and an FOV of 500 mm. The ultra-low dose CT images were reconstructed using AIIR and HIR algorithms, respectively. The attenuation of PET images was corrected by PET-AIIR and PET-HIR, while the standard-dose CT images were reconstructed by HIR. The image quality and quantitative parameters of both the ultra-low-dose CT images and the standard-dose CT images were evaluated and compared.

The results of the analysis showed that, in comparison with the standard-dose CT with HIR, ultra-low-dose CT with AIIR achieved equivalent image quality in the neck, chest, and lower limbs, although the subjective scores decreased in the brain and abdomen. The CT_{mean} of the lesion, neck, chest, abdomen, and pelvis in ultra-low-dose CT with AIIR was equivalent to that in standard-dose CT with HIR, although a significant difference was found in the brain and lower limb skeleton. Additionally, the CT_{sd} of ultra-low-dose CT decreased in the neck muscle, back muscle, mediastinum, liver, lumbar muscle, first lumbar spine, gluteus maximus, lower limb muscle, and lesion. With the exception of the brain, neck, lung, sigmoid colon, and lower limbs, the SNR of the ultra-low-dose CT was higher than that of the standard-does CT, and there was no significant difference in the contrast-to-noise ratio (CNR). Analysis of the attenuation-corrected PET images revealed that compared with those of PET-HIR, the SUV_{max}, SUV_{mean}, and SUV of PET-AIIR remained largely unchanged in the whole body and lesions, and the correlation analysis demonstrated a high degree of consistency of these parameters between the PET-HIR and PET-AIIR ($r > 0.99$).

In this study, it was observed that ultra-low-dose CT-AIIR had poorer image quality in the brain and abdomen, likely because of the positioning of the patient's hands on the sides of the body, which impeded the penetration of high-density X-rays into the skull and bilateral upper limbs. Except in the brain, the CNR of ultra-low-dose CT-AIIR was comparable to that of standard-dose CT-HIR, suggesting that the AIIR algorithm was successful in significantly reducing the noise of ultra-low-dose CT images while maintaining a high CNR. Moreover, after changing the reconstruction algorithm, there was no significant effect on the PET images. Despite the overall quality of the ultra-low-dose CT images being inferior to that of the standard-dose CT images, it is evident that the AIIR algorithm was able to decrease the image noise and increase the SNR.

References

1. Liu G, Chen S, Hu Y, Cao S, Yang X, Zhou Y, et al. Respiratory-gated PET imaging with reduced acquisition time for suspect malignancies: the first experience in application of total-body PET/CT. Eur Radiol. 2023;33(5):3366–76.
2. Walker MD, Morgan AJ, Bradley KM, McGowan DR. Data-driven respiratory gating outperforms device-based gating for clinical ^{18}F-FDG PET/CT. J Nucl Med. 2020;61(11):1678–83.
3. Wagatsuma K, Miwa K, Sakata M, Oda K, Ono H, Kameyama M, et al. Comparison between new-generation SiPM-based and conventional PMT-based TOF-PET/CT. Phys Med. 2017;42:203–10.
4. Ciappuccini R, Desmonts C, Licaj I, Blanc-Fournier C, Bardet S, Aide N. Optimization of a dedicated protocol using a small-voxel PSF reconstruction for head-and-neck ^{18}FDG PET/CT imaging in differentiated thyroid cancer. EJNMMI Res. 2018;8(1):104.
5. Sui X, Tan H, Yu H, Xiao J, Qi C, Cao Y, et al. Exploration of the total-body PET/CT reconstruction protocol with ultra-low ^{18}F-FDG activity over a wide range of patient body mass indices. EJNMMI Phys. 2022;9(1):17.

6. Mehranian A, Wollenweber SD, Walker MD, Bradley KM, Fielding PA, Su KH, et al. Image enhancement of whole-body oncology [^{18}F]-FDG PET scans using deep neural networks to reduce noise. Eur J Nucl Med Mol Imaging. 2022;49(2):539–49.
7. Cherry SR. The 2006 Henry N. Wagner Lecture: of mice and men (and positrons)—advances in PET imaging technology. J Nucl Med. 2006;47(11):1735–45.
8. Shang K, Cui B, Ma J, Shuai D, Liang Z, Jansen F, et al. Clinical evaluation of whole-body oncologic PET with time-of-flight and point-spread function for the hybrid PET/MR system. Eur J Radiol. 2017;93:70–5.
9. Koopman D, van Dalen JA, Lagerweij MC, Arkies H, de Boer J, Oostdijk AH, et al. Improving the detection of small lesions using a state-of-the-art time-of-flight PET/CT system and small-voxel reconstructions. J Nucl Med Technol. 2015;43(1):21–7.
10. Cherry SR, Jones T, Karp JS, Qi J, Moses WW, Badawi RD. Total-body PET: maximizing sensitivity to create new opportunities for clinical research and patient care. J Nucl Med. 2018;59(1):3–12.
11. Cherry SR, Badawi RD, Karp JS, Moses WW, Price P, Jones T. Total-body imaging: transforming the role of positron emission tomography. Sci Transl Med. 2017;9(381):aaf6169.
12. Badawi RD, Shi H, Hu P, Chen S, Xu T, Price PM, et al. First human imaging studies with the EXPLORER total-body PET scanner. J Nucl Med. 2019;60(3):299–303.
13. Adams MC, Turkington TG, Wilson JM, Wong TZ. A systematic review of the factors affecting accuracy of SUV measurements. Am J Roentgenol. 2010;195(2):310–20.
14. Jaskowiak CJ, Bianco JA, Perlman SB, Fine JP. Influence of reconstruction iterations on ^{18}F-FDG PET/CT standardized uptake values. J Nucl Med. 2005;46(3):424–8.
15. Sui X, Liu G, Hu P, Chen S, Yu H, Wang Y, et al. Total-body PET/computed tomography highlights in clinical practice: experiences from Zhongshan Hospital, Fudan University. PET Clin. 2021;16(1):9–14.
16. Watson CC, Casey ME, Bendriem B, Carney JP, Townsend DW, Eberl S, et al. Optimizing injected dose in clinical PET by accurately modeling the counting-rate response functions specific to individual patient scans. J Nucl Med. 2005;46(11):1825–34.
17. Chang T, Chang G, Kohlmyer S, Clark JW, Rohren E, Mawlawi OR. Effects of injected dose, BMI and scanner type on NECR and image noise in PET imaging. Phys Med Biol. 2011;56(16):5275–85.
18. Yang FJ, Ai SY, Wu R, Lv Y, Xie HF, Dong Y, et al. Impact of total variation regularized expectation maximization reconstruction on the image quality of ^{68}Ga-PSMA PET: a phantom and patient study. Br J Radiol. 2021;94(1120):20201356.
19. Prieto E, Garcia-Velloso MJ, Rodriguez-Fraile M, Moran V, Garcia-Garcia B, Guillen F, et al. Significant dose reduction is feasible in FDG PET/CT protocols without compromising diagnostic quality. Phys Med. 2018;46:134–9.
20. Kalra MK, Maher MM, Sahani DV, Blake MA, Hahn PF, Avinash GB, et al. Low-dose CT of the abdomen: evaluation of image improvement with use of noise reduction filters pilot study. Radiology. 2003;228(1):251–6.
21. Leipsic J, Labounty TM, Heilbron B, Min JK, Mancini GB, Lin FY, et al. Adaptive statistical iterative reconstruction: assessment of image noise and image quality in coronary CT angiography. Am J Roentgenol. 2010;195(3):649–54.
22. Kumar S, Pandey AK, Sharma P, Malhotra A, Kumar R. Optimization of the CT acquisition protocol to reduce patient dose without compromising the diagnostic quality for PET-CT: a phantom study. Nucl Med Commun. 2012;33(2):164–70.
23. Bertolini V, Palmieri A, Bassi MC, Bertolini M, Trojani V, Piccagli V, et al. CT protocol optimisation in PET/CT: a systematic review. EJNMMI Phys. 2020;7(1):17.
24. Ho SI, Reece C, Hennessy T, Horsfield M, McBride B. Influence of X-ray computed tomography (CT) exposure and reconstruction parameters on positron emission tomography (PET) quantitation. EJNMMI Phys. 2020;7(1):62.

Interpretation of the Consensus of Oncological ^{18}F-FDG Total-Body PET/CT Imaging

9

Haojun Yu, Yiqiu Zhang, and Hongcheng Shi

On April 22nd, 2019, the world's first total-body positron emission tomography–computed tomography (TB PET/CT) imaging system, uEXPLORER, was installed at Zhongshan Hospital Affiliated to Fudan University. The primary challenge faced by the team, as the first scientific research and clinical application institution to receive this system, was how to maximize the excellent physical performance advantages of this innovative device, fully utilize its application potential, and reasonably expand its applicable fields. Professor Hongcheng Shi, Director of the Department of Nuclear Medicine, Zhongshan Hospital, led the investigation and delved deeper into unfamiliar fields, ranging from clinical validation to scientific investigation and to clinical utilization and promotion. The team's research on image quality, diagnostic accuracy, and clinical feasibility of the device has laid the foundation for the formulation of optimal examination schemes for different clinical application scenarios. Moreover, with the continuous iteration of clinical practice experience, a complete set of operating specifications for TB PET/CT tumor imaging has been formed. Additionally, the team has focused on the characteristics of the equipment, such as low dose, rapid scanning, and dynamic imaging, and conducted a wide range of scientific research. As a result, nearly 20 papers have been published in top journals in the field of imaging medicine, such as the Journal of Nuclear Medicine (JNM), European Journal of Nuclear Medicine and Molecular Imaging (EJNMMI), European Radiology and Chinese Nuclear Medicine and Molecular Imaging Journal, thus laying a solid foundation for the formation of expert consensus. The use of TB PET/CT in China is increasing and its clinical applications are becoming more widespread; therefore, it is essential to share the research and clinical application experience and achievements of the Department of Nuclear Medicine, Zhongshan Hospital with the industry to promote the standardized clinical application of TB PET/CT and benefit the majority of patients. In January 2021, Professor Hongcheng Shi suggested that an expert consensus should be drafted by nuclear medicine experts from various TB PET/CT application institutions in China, who reacted positively and began to organize a team. This would allow them to share their clinical research and exploratory clinical application experience and achievements of the Department of Nuclear Medicine, Zhongshan Hospital with the industry, standardize the clinical application of TB PET/CT, and ultimately benefit most patients.

In 2022, a paper titled "Expert consensus on oncological [18F]FDG total-body PET/CT imaging (Version 1)" was jointly written and published in the internationally authoritative journal *European Radiology* by nuclear medicine experts

H. Yu · Y. Zhang · H. Shi (✉)
Department of Nuclear Medicine, Zhongshan Hospital, Fudan University, Shanghai, China
e-mail: shi.hongcheng@zs-hospital.sh.cn

© Shanghai Scientific and Technical Publishers 2024

H. Shi et al. (eds.), *Total-Body PET/CT*, https://doi.org/10.1007/978-981-97-5065-8_9

from 11 renowned large hospitals in China, led by the Department of Nuclear Medicine, Zhongshan Hospital [1]. These hospitals included Sun Yat-sen University Cancer Center, Henan Provincial People's Hospital, Tongji Hospital affiliated to Huazhong University of Science and Technology, First Hospital Affiliated to Shanxi Medical University, Renji Hospital affiliated to Shanghai Jiaotong University, Ruijin Hospital affiliated to Shanghai Jiaotong University, Nanfang Hospital affiliated to Southern Medical University, The First Affiliated Hospital of Shandong First Medical University, Guangdong Provincial People's Hospital, and the Chinese PLA General Hospital.

This expert consensus serves as the first systematic guidelines for the clinical application of TB PET/CT globally and has been published as a milestone, filling the gap in this field, and promoting the transition of TB PET/CT tumor imaging from scientific research to standardized tumor imaging, thus empowering the clinical application of the resultant images. This expert consensus is structured into two sections: conventional static scanning and dynamic scanning, from the perspectives of process management, patient management, image quality, radiation safety, and patient experience, generally encompassing the protocol process of TB PET/CT, injection dose, scanning time, image reconstruction, and dynamic scanning, as well as many other aspects.

9.1 Definitions

9.1.1 Scope of TB PET/CT Imaging

TB PET/CT imaging offers a distinct advantage over traditional PET/CT in that it provides a total-body image from the skull vertex to toe in a single-bed scan. This is in contrast to traditional PET/CT, which requires multiple bed scans to be combined to create a total-body image from the head to the mid-thigh.

9.1.2 Injection Dose Stratification

The full injection dose is set at 3.7 MBq/kg [2], the low dose or half dose injection is set at 1.85 MBq/kg, and the ultra-low-dose injection is set at 0.37 MBq/kg. Further research is needed to explore the feasibility of other activity levels.

9.1.3 Static PET Scanning

Static PET imaging is acquired within a range of 55–75 min post-injection, by the guidelines and specifications of traditional standard axial field of view (SAFOV) tumor imaging [3]. The semi-quantitative indices such as the standardized uptake value (SUV) are then calculated based on the data. The purpose of rapid scan TB PET/CT static imaging is to generate images of a quality comparable to those of conventional PET/CT scanners, but with a shorter acquisition time.

9.1.4 Dynamic PET Scanning

The dynamic PET scanning begins before the injection and can be continued for up to 60 min, or according to the specific requirements of the study. The data acquired is reconstructed into multiple frames of varying lengths.

9.1.5 CT Scanning

Three types of CT scans can be employed to meet various examination requirements: (1) Scout: an ultra-low-dose planar X-ray imaging to ensure that the patient's entire body is within the scan field of view; (2) Attenuation-correction CT (ACCT): a non-contrast-enhanced low-dose CT scan to correct photon attenuation; and (3) Diagnostic CT: a full-dose CT scan to meet diagnostic requirements. Different tube currents may be selected according to different parts of the body. It is recommended that head and trunk CT scans can be performed separately with the corresponding parameters, and contrast-enhanced CT scans can be performed according to clinical needs.

9.2 Routine TB PET/CT Static Scanning

The routine protocol for ^{18}F-fluorodeoxyglucose (FDG) TB PET/CT static scanning is comparable to that of conventional PET/CT. However, our experience has revealed certain distinctions between the two modalities. These distinctions include the management of claustrophobic patients, the dosage of medication, the duration of acquisition, and the sequence of PET and CT scans.

9.2.1 Personalization of the Scanning Protocol

The sequence of PET/CT scans is as follows: CT Scout, ACCT, PET, and diagnostic CT. The extent of coverage of the diagnostic CT is determined based on the data obtained from the CT Scout, ACCT, and PET images. The scanning sequence and the injection dose can be personalized based on the patient's condition. For patients with tumors who are unable to remain motionless for an extended time, it is recommended to use a full-dose rapid scan. It is also feasible to prioritize the completion of the diagnostic CT scan after ascertaining the scan range based on the CT scout images and prior imaging data.

The selection of oral or intravenous agents for contrast-enhanced CT scans must be conducted following established protocols. The physician should carefully consider the indications, contraindications, and potential drug interactions associated with the contrast agent before its administration.

The utilization of TB PET/CT (uEXPLORER) is advantageous because of its AFOV of up to 194 cm. However, such scanning might cause distress in patients who are predisposed to claustrophobia. Based on our experience, the utilization of TB PET/CT does not necessarily lead to more claustrophobia among patients compared with conventional PET/CT, despite the longer axial scan bore. Occasionally, clinicians might be confronted with claustrophobic patients. In such cases, it is essential to consider the implementation of the appropriate solution, such as sedation, if necessary. The low-dose or ultra-low-dose protocols in pediatric patients have significant clinical implications. The TB PET/CT scanner has enabled the implementation of such protocols, thereby allowing for the acquisition of optimal image quality while minimizing radiation exposure.

9.2.2 Quality Control

Before use, TB PET/CT scanners must undergo corresponding quality control for the CT and PET components. Daily quality control includes CT tube preheating and PET source-less calibration, which involves using ^{176}Lu as the radiation source for daily quality control in the detector. Weekly quality control includes CT air calibration and PET source calibration.

TB PET/CT imaging systems have an ultra-high sensitivity, resulting in large raw data files. The size of the data is dependent on the injection dose and the acquisition time. For full-dose static acquisition, the size of the raw data is approximately 40–50 Gb (calculated with an injection dose of 6.6 mCi and an acquisition time of 5 min), while a conventional static PET acquisition is approximately 3–4 Gb (calculated with an injection dose of 6.4 mCi, 5-bed acquisitions, and 2 min per bed acquisition). This is a ten-fold difference; hence, it is necessary to check the disk space of the reconstruction computer before PET acquisition to avoid any issues.

9.2.3 TB PET/CT Imaging Acquisition and Processing

9.2.3.1 Injection Dose

The administration of ^{18}F-FDG can be reduced to low (1.85 MBq/kg) or ultra-low (0.37 MBq/kg) doses with similar quality as the full dose

(3.7 MBq/kg). This allows for personalized imaging protocols for each patient. The injection dose and acquisition time can be adjusted according to the body mass index (BMI) of the patient [4]. TB PET/CT has a greater acquisition efficiency than conventional PET/CT, allowing full-dose injection to reduce the PET acquisition time to 30–45 s. To ensure optimal image quality and operational efficiency, close attention should be paid to the time interval between ^{18}F-FDG administration and scanning.

9.2.3.2 Patient Position

The patient's position is adjusted according to the location of the lesion to avoid artifacts. The arms can be raised to reduce artifacts in the abdomen and pelvis. For brain CT imaging, it is recommended to place the arms by the side of the body. This might cause CT truncation artifacts; however, this can be improved using the adaptive filter preset in the system and by extending the reconstruction FOV to 700 mm.

9.2.3.3 Scanning Procedure

The standard protocol involves CT scout, low-dose ACCT, TB PET, optional diagnostic body CT, diagnostic head CT, or contrast-enhanced CT. The imaging sequence of conventional PET/CT is fixed, while the imaging sequence of TB PET/CT can be adjusted to optimize diagnostic efficiency. If the patient is in unbearable pain, a non-contrast CT scan can be performed first, followed by PET imaging. For patients who experience displacement during the examination, PET images from the first 30–45 s can be reconstructed, or divided into several short-time images, from which images that meet the diagnostic requirements can be selected. If necessary, contrast-enhanced CT is recommended after PET scanning. The range of diagnostic CT scanning can be adjusted according to clinical needs, and ACCT can be used instead of diagnostic CT under certain special circumstances.

9.2.3.4 Acquisition Settings

1. **CT Acquisition settings**

   The CT acquisition settings are not associated with the injection dose of radiotracer. For scout scans, it is recommended to employ 80–120 kV, 20–40 mA for adults, and 70–80 kV, 20 mA for children. Attenuation correction CT settings are recommended to be 120 kV, 5–20 mA, 40 mm collimation width, 0.98–1.3 pitch, and 0.5–0.8 s rotation time. The recommended settings for diagnostic body CT parameters are 120 kV, with the tube current using modulation technology, 40 mm collimation width, 0.9625 pitch, and 0.5 s rotation time, while diagnostic head CT settings are recommended to be 120 kV, 280 mA, 20 mm collimation width, 0.6750 pitch, and 0.8 s rotation time.
2. **Full-dose PET acquisition time**

   The recommended scan time for a routine scan is 0.5–2 min, and 0.5–1 min for a rapid scan [5–7]. Prolonging the scan time appropriately (e.g., 5 min) can result in improved image quality.
3. **Low-dose PET acquisition time**

   The recommended scan time for a routine scan is 3–5 min, and 2–4 min for a rapid scan [8, 9].
4. **Ultra-low-dose PET acquisition time**

   The recommended scan time for a routine scan is 7–15 min and 6–8 min for a rapid scan [10, 11].

9.2.3.5 PET Reconstruction

PET reconstruction settings for PET data should be adjusted to meet the standards or guidelines, such as the quantitative evaluation standards approved by the European Association of Nuclear Medicine Research Ltd. (EARL), and the point spread function (PSF) for visual evaluation standards. The manufacturer's options should be consulted when selecting different reconstruction settings. The recommended reconstruction settings for a body scan are as follows: 192 × 192 matrix, ordered subset expectation maximization (OSEM) (3 iterations, 20 subsets) with attenuation, scatter, random, and normalization correction, and a time-of-flight (TOF) option should be applied to all reconstruction settings. For head reconstruction, the settings are as follows: 192 × 192 matrix, OSEM (3 iterations, 20 subsets) with attenuation, scatter, random, and normalization correction. The matrix size can be adjusted to achieve a balance between reconstruction time and spatial resolution, according to the clinical requirements.

9.2.3.6 Diagnostic CT Reconstruction

The recommended reconstruction settings for body CT are as follows: 1 mm slice thickness, 1 mm slice interval, 512 × 512 matrix, and 500 mm FOV. Head reconstruction settings are as follows: 2 mm slice thickness, 2 mm slice interval, 512 × 512 matrix, and 300 mm FOV. Particular attention should be paid to the brain, for which the reconstruction slice thickness might be reduced to less than 2 mm.

9.3 TB PET/CT Dynamic Scanning

^{18}F-FDG TB PET/CT dynamic scanning has important value in tumor diagnosis, prognosis, and survival prediction, and further valuable diagnostic information can be obtained through pharmacokinetic analysis. Compared with traditional PET, TB PET has ultra-high sensitivity and can obtain higher temporal resolution and higher signal-to-noise ratio of the blood input function, thus achieving more accurate tracer kinetic analysis.

9.3.1 Quality Control

The daily and weekly quality control required is similar to those of the TB PET/CT static scan. Particular emphasis should be placed on the dynamic acquisition process for an extended period (≥60 min). The prolonged period without utilizing CT means that the thermal capacity of the tube will be further diminished, necessitating preheating of the thermal capacity of the tube to greater than 15% before starting the scan, otherwise it might result in an inability to employ higher parameters for diagnostic CT scanning.

Before initiating a TB PET dynamic scan, it is necessary to ensure that the residual storage capacity of the reconstruction computer is sufficient to accommodate the dynamic acquisition, to avoid premature termination of the dynamic acquisition caused by inadequate storage space. The raw data from dynamic PET acquisition necessitates a substantial storage capacity, estimated to be approximately 800 Gb (calculated based on an injection dose of 7 mCi and an acquisition time of 60 min), thus necessitating stringent data storage and management.

9.3.2 Precautions During Acquisition

9.3.2.1 Patient Positioning

It is recommended that the patient be positioned feet-first, with the headrest replaced by an extension plate to facilitate intravenous injection in the foot. The arms should be placed at the side of the body. For patients with a compulsive position, their position can be adjusted accordingly with the aid of cushions to ensure the patient is in the most comfortable position during the acquisition process.

9.3.2.2 Injection Site

Foot intravenous injection is preferred for convenience. Intravenous injection at the elbow vein is a viable option for patients with their arms up. When the foot vein is difficult to access, elbow vein injection may be used as an alternative using a 1-m long extension tube to facilitate the injection. It is important to note that the use of an extension tube might impact the count rate and the image quality of dynamic PET imaging. It is advised to keep the foot warm before the patient enters the scanning room to avoid vasoconstriction, which would impede venous injection.

9.3.2.3 Injection Procedure

It is recommended to establish a venous channel on the back of the foot and inject a small amount of saline to confirm the successful establishment of the channel. Bolus injection should be performed immediately after image acquisition begins, followed by a saline flush (Fig. 9.1). The efficacy of the dynamic scanning process is contingent upon the collaborative effort between the

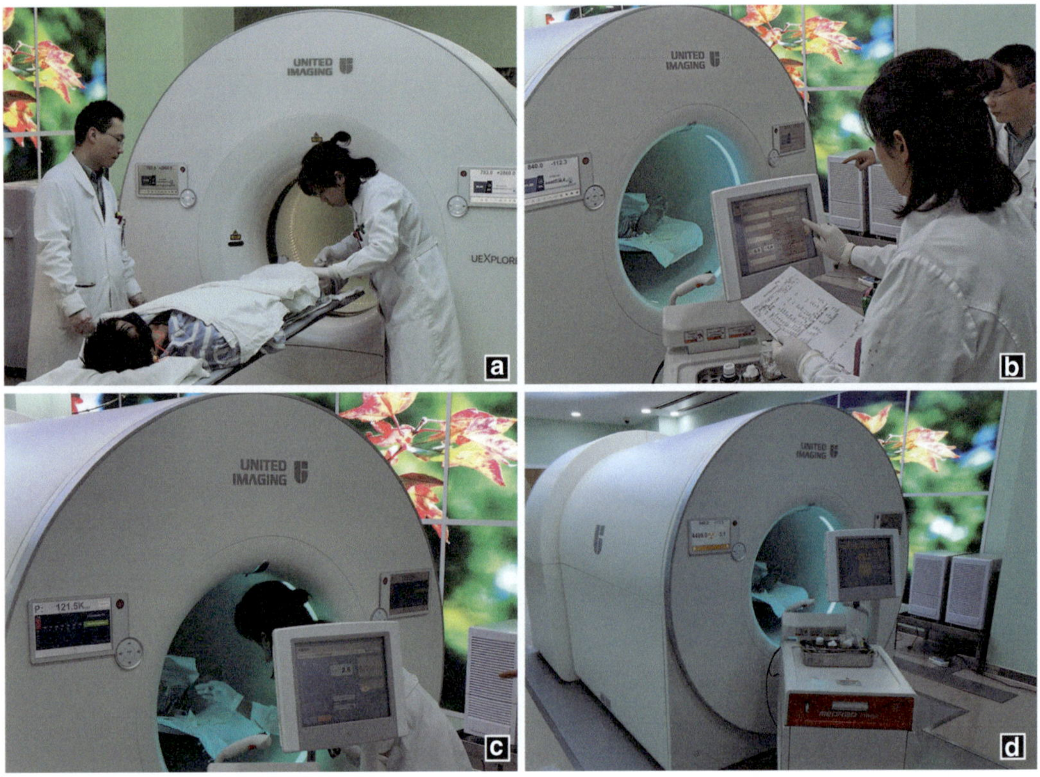

Fig. 9.1 Tracer injection process of TB PET/CT dynamic scanning. (**a**) Establishing an intravenous channel; (**b**) Determining the injection dose; (**c**) Testing the patency of the injection channel; (**d**) Bolus injection

technician and the nurse, because this might affect the quality of the dynamic data. For example, if the PET acquisition starts after the bolus injection, the dynamic information might be lost. The implementation of an automated syringe cart is strongly advocated for dynamic imaging because it can provide greater precision, reduce the potential for errors, and enhance the quality of dynamic scan data.

9.3.3 PET/CT Image Acquisition and Processing

9.3.3.1 Scanning Procedure

The dynamic scanning comprises CT Scout, ACCT, PET, and diagnostic CT for the body and head. The acquisition sequence can be adjusted according to the patient's medical history and examination purpose. For instance, to assess the efficacy of therapeutic interventions in neoplastic and pediatric patients, low-dose computed tomography (CT) scanning is generally sufficient to meet the clinical requirements.

9.3.3.2 Setting Parameters

The parameters for CT Scout, low-dose ACCT, and diagnostic CT are similar to those of the routine PET/CT scan. The selection of the injection dose of the radiotracer can be made between a full dose, a low dose, or an ultra-low dose. Dynamic PET imaging is typically recommended to be acquired for 60 min; however, the duration might vary depending on the purpose of the study.

9.3.3.3 PET Reconstruction

The selection of various imaging frame modes and the configuration of different frame durations, with the shortest being 100 ms/frame, is feasible. These settings are primarily determined based on the purpose of the examination. The frames are recommended as 36 frames × 5 s/frame and 19 frames ×

180 s/frame. The following frame schemes can also be adapted for 60 min dynamic PET data: 30 frames × 2 s/frame, 12 frames × 5 s/frame, 6 frames × 10 s/frame, 4 frames × 30 s/frame, 25 frames × 60 s/frame, and 15 frames × 120 s/frame. A shorter frame duration might introduce bias, thus necessitating the selection of alternative reconstruction schemes with longer frame durations. The matrix size, slice thickness, number of iterations, number of subsets, and FOV can be adjusted to accommodate particular circumstances. Corrections such as attenuation, scattering, randomization, and normalization can be applied to further refine the reconstruction settings. The injection dose can be taken into consideration when optimizing the aforementioned parameters.

9.3.3.4 Challenges

As experience in dynamic imaging increases, the majority of reconstruction parameters are based on the manufacturer's recommendations. As the number of dynamic scans increases further advances will be pinpointed. Patient cooperation is essential, because motion artifacts or early termination of dynamic acquisition might occur. Therefore, pre-acquisition assessment and patient cooperation are crucial and should be undertaken. Further advances in patient immobilization and pre-scan coaching are necessary to prevent voluntary patient movement. Negative-pressure vacuum bags and blankets are recommended to ensure patient comfort. Dynamic PET imaging necessitates the patient spend a longer time in the scanner. To reduce patients' waiting time, continual optimization and dynamic adjustment of operational and managerial processes are necessary. The time interval between injection and scanning must also be precisely regulated to minimize the effect of dynamic acquisition on static acquisition. Recent studies have sought to reduce the duration of total-body parameter imaging via PET scans [12–14]. Maximizing the efficiency of the most sophisticated TB PET/CT scanner necessitates further investigation and refinement.

References

1. Yu H, Gu Y, Fan W, et al. Expert consensus on oncological [^{18}F]FDG total-body PET/CT imaging (version 1). Eur Radiol. 2023;33(1):615–26.
2. Delbeke D, Coleman RE, Guiberteau MJ, et al. Procedure guideline for tumor imaging with ^{18}F-FDG PET/CT 1.0. J Nucl Med. 2006;47(5):885–95.
3. Quantitative FDG-PET Technical Committee. UPICT oncology FDG-PET CT protocol. https://qibawiki.rsna.org/index.php/FDG-PET_Biomarker_Ctte.
4. Xiao J, Yu H, Sui X, et al. Can the BMI-based dose regimen be used to reduce injection activity and to obtain a constant image quality in oncological patients by ^{18}F-FDG total-body PET/CT imaging? Eur J Nucl Med Mol Imaging. 2021;49(1):269–78.
5. Zhang YQ, Hu PC, Wu R, et al. The image quality, lesion detectability, and acquisition time of ^{18}F-FDG total-body PET/CT in oncological patients. Eur J Nucl Med Mol Imaging. 2020;47(11):2507–15.
6. Hu P, Zhang Y, Yu H, et al. Total-body ^{18}F-FDG PET/CT scan in oncology patients: how fast could it be? Eur J Nucl Med Mol Imaging. 2021;48(8):2384–94.
7. Hu Y, Liu G, Yu H, et al. Diagnostic performance of total-body ^{18}F-FDG PET/CT with fast 2-min acquisition for liver tumours: comparison with conventional PET/CT. Eur J Nucl Med Mol Imaging. 2022;49(10):3538–46.
8. Tan H, Sui X, Yin H, et al. Total-body PET/CT using half-dose FDG and compared with conventional PET/CT using full-dose FDG in lung cancer. Eur J Nucl Med Mol Imaging. 2021;48(6):1966–75.
9. He Y, Gu Y, Yu H, et al. Optimizing acquisition times for total-body positron emission tomography/computed tomography with half-dose ^{18}F-fluorodeoxyglucose in oncology patients. EJNMMI Phys. 2022;9(1):45.
10. Tan H, Cai D, Sui X, et al. Investigating ultra-low-dose total-body [^{18}F]-FDG PET/CT in colorectal cancer: initial experience. Eur J Nucl Med Mol Imaging. 2021;49(3):1002–11.
11. Hu Y, Liu G, Yu H, et al. Feasibility of acquisitions using total-body PET/CT with an ultra-low 18F-FDG activity. J Nucl Med. 2022;63(6):959–65.
12. Liu G, Yu H, Shi D, et al. Short-time total-body dynamic PET imaging performance in quantifying the kinetic metrics of ^{18}F-FDG in healthy volunteers. Eur J Nucl Med Mol Imaging. 2022;49(8):2493–503.
13. Wu Y, Feng T, Zhao Y, et al. Whole-body parametric imaging of ^{18}F-FDG PET using uEXPLORER with reduced scanning time. J Nucl Med. 2022;63(4):622–8.
14. Feng T, Zhao Y, Shi H, et al. Total-body quantitative parametric imaging of early kinetics of ^{18}F-FDG. J Nucl Med. 2021;62(5):738–44.

10 Recommended Workflow of Total-Body PET/CT Application in Clinical

Guobing Liu, Yiqiu Zhang, Yushen Gu, Haojun Yu, and Hongcheng Shi

The capabilities of total-body positron emission tomography–computed tomography (TB PET/CT) surpass those of conventional short-axis PET/CT, offering a variety of imaging options, such as half-dose or ultra-low (1/10) dose scanning, rapid scanning, and ultra-long time-delay static imaging, as well as TB real-time dynamic scanning. To maximize the performance of the equipment and better meet clinical needs, as well as accommodate the requirements of clinical research, it is essential to have a scientifically and reasonably arranged workflow. If the patient's examination is arranged in real time on site, with a comprehensive evaluation of the patient beforehand, then the workflow can be more easily realized. However, if some patients are selected in real time from those who arrive for examination on the same day for TB PET/CT examination, then workflow optimization becomes challenging. Nevertheless, regardless of whether it is an appointment system or a temporary arrangement, ensuring a smooth and high-quality process, as well as close cooperation between each part of the process, is important to promote efficient operation.

10.1 Construction of an Efficient TB PET/CT Operating System

The complexity of the TB PET/CT examination process has increased with the availability of multiple options (Fig. 10.1). This complexity is further compounded when multiple PET/CTs are operated simultaneously (Fig. 10.2). At our center, four PET/CTs are operated in parallel, with approximately 100 patients examined daily, mostly comprising walk-ins and complete examinations on the same day. Patients with the greatest potential benefit are selected for TB PET/CT examination based on their medical history. For those selected for TB PET/CT examination, the dynamic or static collection is chosen based on the patient's condition, as well as the appropriate injection dose and the corresponding collection time. This process is highly interconnected, with real-time information exchange enabled by the "Intelligence Center" responsible for overall coordination, thus allowing for the efficient operation of the entire system.

The "Intelligent Center" is responsible for organizing patient examinations in accordance

G. Liu · Y. Zhang · Y. Gu · H. Yu · H. Shi (✉)
Department of Nuclear Medicine, Zhongshan Hospital, Fudan University, Shanghai, China
e-mail: shi.hongcheng@zs-hospital.sh.cn

© Shanghai Scientific and Technical Publishers 2024
H. Shi et al. (eds.), *Total-Body PET/CT*, https://doi.org/10.1007/978-981-97-5065-8_10

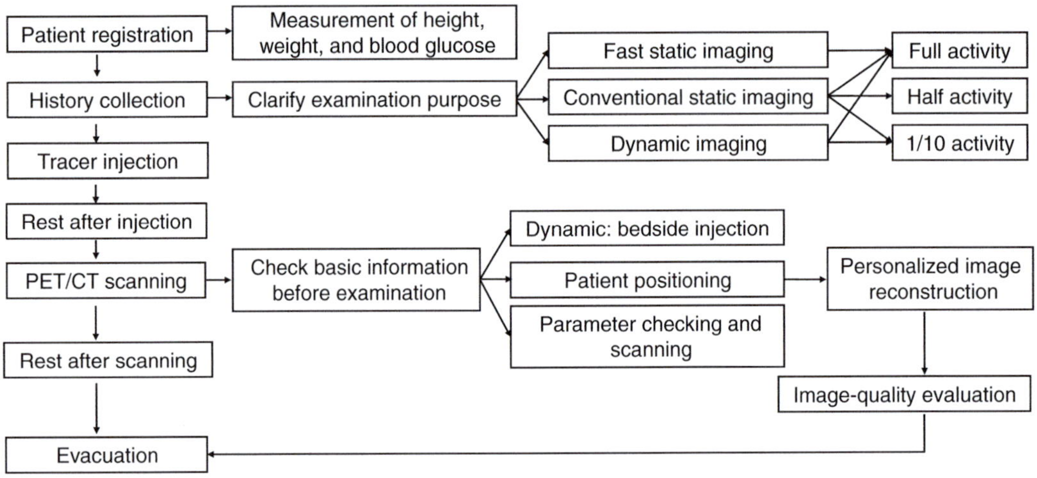

Fig. 10.1 Schematic diagram of the process of TB PET/CT examination

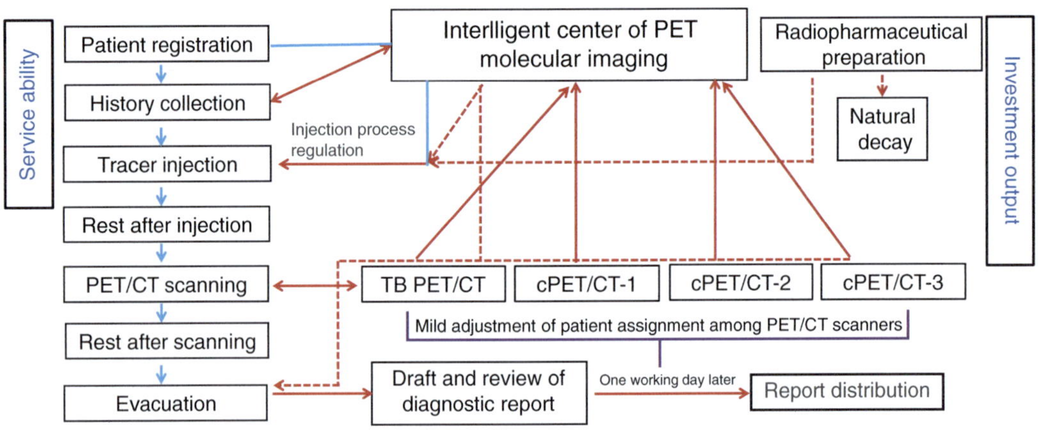

Fig. 10.2 Schematic diagram of the workflow for simultaneous running of the four PET/CT scanners in the Department of Nuclear Medicine, Zhongshan Hospital

with standard protocols. By exchanging real-time information with each step of the workflow, the Center can adjust and optimize the process promptly, thus ensuring maximized entire working efficiency.

10.2 Case Study of Efficient Operation of TB PET/CT

In the field of nuclear medicine, TB PET/CT has emerged as a multi-modal imaging technique that can be tailored to meet individual patient needs. In clinical practice, especially when dealing with a high volume of patient examinations, there is often a need to balance the requirements of routine clinical work and clinical research. To ensure the quality of service, it is necessary to complete the examinations of many patients quickly, while also minimizing the use of radiotracers and adhering to a standardized examination process. To achieve optimal overall operational efficiency, it is essential to develop a combination of examination sequences for patients with different needs.

At the PET/CT Molecular Imaging Center of Zhongshan Hospital, more than 100 people are examined daily, with the majority being patients with tumors, including children, interspersed with examinations of non-tumor patients, as well as multi-tracer imaging and dynamic imaging. To optimize the workflow, it is necessary to solve key problems and appropriately optimize and combine sorting examinations, cross-arrange dynamic scans, fast scans, low-dose or ultra-low-dose scans, and combination scans involving multi-tracers. During clinical application, the main challenges faced by TB PET/CT examination can be categorized as follows:

10.2.1 A Large Number of Patients Awaiting Examination

Given an adequate amount of radiotracer, full-dose injection and rapid scanning can alleviate the pressure of a backlog of patients awaiting examination. When patients have personalized needs, such as half-dose or ultra-low-dose scanning, it is recommended that they are scheduled as late as possible, because lower injection doses necessitate longer acquisition times. Scheduling these patients at the beginning of the queue will not be effective in quickly reducing the backlog.

10.2.2 Limited Amount of Radiotracer

Under a fixed injection dose, it is suggested to inject the full dose, or the upper limit of the dose recommended by the guidelines at an early stage to meet the inspection needs of as many patients as possible, while minimizing the loss caused by radioactive nuclide decay. Fast scanning should also be used to complete a certain number of patient inspections with a relatively sufficient radiotracer dose. When the amount of radiotracer is not sufficient in the later stage, it is suggested to select the half dose and ultra-low dose in turn, and the acquisition time should be increased to meet the requirement for more patient inspections.

For example, on one day of June 2022, the center only had a total of 21,978 MBq (594 mCi) of ^{18}F-FDG but expected to complete many patient examinations (Table 10.1). A total of 29 patient examinations were completed within 9 h using a combination of ultra-long dynamic scanning, full-dose rapid scanning, and low-dose or ultra-low-dose scanning. Radiotracer injection of the first patient was performed at the bedside and dynamic scanning was conducted for 60 min to meet clinical and research needs. Subsequent injections were administered in sequence, transitioning from high dose to low dose, with a 65 ± 10 min post-injection waiting time and cumulative machine occupancy time from completion of the examination to leaving the machine. The PET acquisition for full-dose injection was 5 min, including the machine occupancy time, with each patient taking 10–12 min. The eighth case was a follow-up, using the same half-dose injection scheme as the previous examination, with a PET acquisition time of 10 min and 15–18 min of machine occupancy. Six cases were clinical research injection schemes, with a standard 5.55 MBq/kg injection and 10 min of PET acquisition. The 19th patient was injected with a 1/10 dose.

10.2.3 Examination According to Diverse Requirements

The concept of diverse requirements comprises various injection doses and types of radiotracers for dynamic and static imaging. The dynamic acquisition is typically arranged at the first or last session, and when the demand increases, the appropriate time for dynamic acquisition is chosen based on the availability of radiotracers and the number of patients to be examined. When the requirements of both routine clinical scans and scientific research coexist, prioritizing clinical research projects facilitates the attainment of higher-quality research outcomes.

On one day of January 2022, the supply of radiotracers was sufficient, although the personalized examination scheme for the patients to be examined was complex. TB PET/CT was completed for 17 patients in approximately 13 h, including seven dynamic collections (three patients underwent a full-dose, 60-min scan; one patient underwent a half-dose, 75-min scan; two patients underwent a 1.11 MBq/kg dose, 60 min

Table 10.1 Completion of the maximum number of patient examinations with limited dose of radiotracer

Patient no	Sex	Age (year)	Type of imaging	Dose (MBq/kg)	Weight (kg)	BMI (kg/m^2)	Injected dose (MBq)	Injection time	Start time[a]	PET acquisition duration (min)
1	Female	59	Dynamic	0.37	53.8	19.1	21.8	8:59	8:52	60
2	Female	65	Static	3.70	62.1	25.2	213.5	9:09	10:04	5
3	Female	53	Static	5.55	56.0	22.4	284.9	9:12	10:26	10
4	Female	42	Static	5.55	49.6	19.6	262.0	9:37	10:40	10
5	Female	66	Static	3.70	53.5	20.1	186.9	9:54	10:57	5
6	Male	60	Static	5.55	78.9	29.0	412.6	10:02	11:14	10
7	Female	46	Static	3.70	70.0	26.7	254.9	10:15	11:30	5
8	Male	39	Static	1.85	71.9	24.6	133.2	10:34	11:41	10
9	Male	67	Static	3.70	78.0	25.8	314.5	10:42	12:02	5
10	Male	65	Static	3.70	76.0	26.0	259.7	9:56	12:13	5
11	Female	34	Static	3.70	64.0	24.4	242.4	10:55	12:28	5
12	Male	68	Static	3.70	77.6	25.3	268.3	11:07	12:43	5
13	Female	60	Static	3.70	52.5	20.5	195.7	11:35	12:54	5
14	Female	71	Static	3.70	37.3	13.7	138.8	12:09	13:04	5
15	Female	65	Static	5.55	58.3	23.7	324.5	12:23	13:14	10
16	Female	57	Static	3.70	49.0	20.9	186.1	12:57	13:52	5
17	Male	56	Static	5.55	66.9	22.9	372.2	12:29	14:02	10
18	Male	76	Static	5.55	56.5	22.7	315.2	13:13	14:16	10
19	Male	69	Dynamic	0.37	80.0	27.7	29.2	14:38	14:39	60
20	Male	62	Static	3.70	63.7	23.2	226.8	14:41	15:46	5
21	Male	73	Static	3.70	64.0	23.3	241.2	14:55	15:56	5
22	Male	69	Static	1.85	79.4	26.8	145.8	15:05	16:05	10
23	Male	67	Static	1.85	61.0	22.4	109.2	15:13	16:19	10
24	Male	66	Static	1.85	72.7	24.9	134.7	15:28	16:32	10
25	Male	60	Static	1.85	62.3	22.1	109.2	16:00	16:50	10
26	Male	54	Static	1.85	87.5	27.6	146.9	16:10	17:05	10
27	Male	66	Static	1.85	65.3	21.1	124.7	16:21	17:18	10
28	Female	65	Static	1.85	50.6	21.1	85.8	16:29	17:34	10
29	Female	43	Static	0.37	78.0	27.6	36.7	16:43	17:48	15

[a] The initial time when the patient started to occupy the machine

scan; one patient underwent an ultra-low dose, 75-min scan) and 2 full-dose and 8 half-dose TB PET/CT static collections (Table 10.2).

In one day of July 2022, two dual-tracer dynamic imaging scans (Table 10.3) were completed in our center. In the center, 33,522 MBq (906 mCi) ^{18}F-FDG was synthesized; however, because of a decrease in Ge-Ga generator capacity, only one batch of ^{68}Ga-fibroblast-activation protein inhibitor (FAPI) was produced in the morning and afternoon, respectively. Twenty-seven patients received a complete TB PET/CT examination in approximately 10 h, including three cases of sub-dynamic scanning (one case received a half-dose, 60-min ^{18}F-FDG scan; two cases underwent an immediate 1.11 MBq/kg ^{68}Ga-FAPI 60 min scan after 15 min of static collection at 1 h).

In clinical practice, especially under the premise of clinical exploratory research, demands are often diverse, complex, and full of uncertainty. To address these real-time demands, TB PET has the advantage of optimizing efficiency, providing a flexible workflow, and striving to fully meet demand. This center provides an important reference for the overall process optimization under different circumstances, based on the above-mentioned principles and the preliminary exploration of high-load instantaneous workflow optimization in non-appointment situations.

Table 10.2 Statistics of patient information of one daily examination that focused mainly on dynamic imaging

Patient no	Sex	Age (year)	Type of imaging	Dose (MBq/kg)	Weight (kg)	BMI (kg/m^2)	Injection dose (MBq)	Injection time	Start time[a]	PET acquisition duration (min)
1	Male	62	Dynamic	1.11	77.7	25.1	99.2	6:58	6:50	60
2	Male	50	Static	1.85	70.0	23.7	140.6	7:08	8:07	10
3	Female	69	Static	3.70	40.0	15.6	162.8	7:38	8:36	5
4	Female	33	Static	1.85	62.5	24.4	127.7	8:10	8:58	10
5	Male	9	Static	1.85	24.5	12.7	51.8	7:12	9:18	10
6	Male	37	Static	1.85	85.0	28.4	173.9	8:43	9:46	10
7	Male	59	Static	1.85	71.4	27.2	144.3	9:01	10:10	10
8	Male	47	Dynamic	1.85	74.0	24.4	129.5	10:40	10:35	75
9	Male	79	Static	3.70	50.0	20.3	185.4	11:30	12:33	5
10	Male	65	Dynamic	3.70	77.5	23.4	284.9	13:05	12:45	60
11	Female	58	Static	1.85	55.0	22.6	111.0	13:18	14:12	10
12	Male	70	Static	1.85	58.0	21.3	109.9	13:34	14:32	10
13	Male	64	Dynamic	1.11	80.0	26.7	101.8	14:55	14:49	60
14	Female	73	Static	1.85	44.0	18.8	86.2	15:16	16:15	10
15	Male	54	Dynamic	0.37	71.5	25.9	27.8	16:44	16:31	75
16	Male	78	Dynamic	3.70	58.0	20.5	214.2	18:14	18:05	60
17	Male	57	Dynamic	3.70	68.5	24.0	269.7	19:27	19:14	60

[a] The initial time when the patient started to occupy the device

Table 10.3 Statistics of patient information of one daily PET/CT examination that contained both multiple radiotracer imaging and dynamic imaging

Patient no	Sex	Age (year)	Type of imaging	Dose (MBq/kg)	Weight (kg)	BMI (kg/m^2)	Injection dose (MBq)	Injection time	Start time[a]	PET acquisition duration (min)
1	Male	67	Dynamic	1.85	82.0	28.0	166.5	7:17	7:08	60
2	Male	27	Static	3.70	70.0	23.9	260.9	7:26	8:21	5
3	Male	70	Static	1.85	64.9	24.1	126.5	7:42	8:33	10
4	Female	70	Static	3.70	33.0	15.7	133.2	7:57	8:51	5
5	Female	32	Static[b]	0.37	53.0	19.7	22.1	7:30	9:14	15
			Dynamic[c]	1.11	53.0	19.7	49.2	9:46	9:46	60
6	Female	64	Static	5.55	75.2	30.1	431.8	9:55	10:48	10
7	Male	81	Static	3.70	68.5	25.8	281.2	10:08	11:05	5
8	Male	57	Static	3.70	63.1	20.6	255.3	10:15	11:16	5
9	Female	66	Static	3.70	72.6	26.7	277.9	10:06	11:30	5
10	Male	73	Static	3.70	75.0	28.9	277.5	10:55	11:41	5
11	Male	84	Static[d]	0.74	68.5	27.4	54.7	9:38	11:53	20
12	Female	69	Static	3.70	44.8	18.6	165.0	11:08	12:23	5
13	Male	67	Static	1.85	61.3	20.0	119.5	10:21	12:36	10
14	Male	59	Static	3.70	60.2	20.3	219.8	11:36	12:57	5
15	Female	55	Static	3.70	54.0	23.1	197.2	11:59	13:08	5
16	Female	65	Static	3.70	56.6	22.1	208.3	12:11	13:19	5
17	Female	66	Static	3.70	41.7	18.5	155.4	12:28	13:30	5
18	Male	59	Static	3.70	67.5	22.8	249.0	12:48	13:43	5
19	Male	41	Static	5.55	80.0	25.8	447.7	13:06	13:56	10
20	Male	59	Static	1.85	83.0	28.1	162.8	13:38	14:39	10
21	Male	78	Static	3.70	64.5	23.7	245.7	13:56	14:56	5
22	Female	51	Static[b]	0.37	55.0	21.0	21.0	13:30	15:13	15
			Dynamic[c]	1.11	55.0	21.0	51.7	15:41	15:41	60

(continued)

Table 10.3 (continued)

Patient no	Sex	Age (year)	Type of imaging	Dose (MBq/kg)	Weight (kg)	BMI (kg/m^2)	Injection dose (MBq)	Injection time	Start time[a]	PET acquisition duration (min)
23	Female	51	Static	1.85	45.0	17.1	88.8	15:58	16:46	10
24	Male	61	Static	1.85	59.1	21.7	114.3	16:09	17:02	10
25	Male	44	Static[d]	0.74	61.0	21.4	49.5	15:29	17:19	20
26	Male	66	Static	0.37	68.0	22.0	27.4	16:20	17:44	15
27	Male	57	Static	0.37	91.5	28.6	34.3	17:00	18:08	15

[a] The initial time of patient occupancy of the equipment
[b] The standard dose is 0.37 MBq/kg of ^{18}F-FDG for static imaging
[c] The standard dose is 1.11 MBq/kg of ^{68}Ga-FAPI for dynamic imaging
[d] Static imaging of ^{68}Ga-FAPI

Postscript

Under the strategic framework of "Zhongshan-United Imaging Healthcare (UIH)," I am deeply honored to lead the team exploring the world's first total-body PET/CT for clinical pre-testing, clinical verification, and clinical application. During this process, I have experienced challenges, opportunities, hard work, and joy. We thank the host hospital and acknowledge the guidance and assistance of our colleagues. We have achieved remarkable results in the 4 years of clinical exploration and application. I would like to express my sincere thanks to:

Professor Jia Fan, who is the academician of Chinese Academy of Sciences and the President of Zhongshan Hospital, for his astute decision to form a strategic alliance with the burgeoning UIH. This has enabled the Department of Nuclear Medicine to become the "pioneer" in the clinical verification and clinical application of numerous molecular imaging equipment manufactured by UIH and to gain experience and make progress in the face of various challenges.

Mr. Qunren Zhang, the director of the General Affairs Department, and his team for their hard work in surmounting numerous obstacles and completing the load-bearing reinforcement and expansion of the total-body PET/CT room, which weighed up to 12 tons and was 10 m long, in approximately 3 weeks. Additionally, I am thankful to the UIH team for their prompt response. The combined efforts of both sides meant that all the tasks from room renovation to equipment installation and commissioning were accomplished in only 1 month.

The Department of Nuclear Medicine for creating the necessary conditions for the clinical implementation of total-body PET/CT while simultaneously managing their busy clinical workload, through the integration and collaboration of "medical, technical, nursery, medicine, and labour."

I am also thankful to all the colleagues in the department for their support in enabling the successful completion of our exploratory work. I would like to express my appreciation to Doctors Guobing Liu, Hui Tan, Yiqiu Zhang, Pengcheng Hu, Yan Hu, and Jie Xiao for their tireless efforts. I am also thankful to my doctoral research students Xiuli Sui, Chi Qi, and Danjie Cai and my master's research students Yanyan Cao, Xueqi Chen, Yibo He, Dilibire Adili, and Runjun Yang, for their exploration of the clinical application of total-body PET/CT and for the successful completion of their studies. I would also like to take this opportunity to remember that during the Chinese New Year of 2022, due to the pandemic breakout, our team stayed up late into the night discussing research topics. I am also thankful to Haojun Yu, the supervisor technician, for his hard work in data management and image processing, which has been instrumental in the exploration of clinical applications, and to Shuguang Chen, the deputy director technician, for his high-quality daily maintenance of the equipment. I would also like to thank the UIH team for their technical support. It is through everyone's concerted efforts, perseverance, and tireless pursuit and exploration that we have achieved these results. Total-body PET/CT is a complex concept of great depth, and its continued exploration and application will require sustained effort over the long term. We are confident that our team will continue to produce sustained output.

© Shanghai Scientific and Technical Publishers 2024
H. Shi et al. (eds.), *Total-Body PET/CT*, https://doi.org/10.1007/978-981-97-5065-8

I am deeply grateful to my family for their unwavering support of my work. Their tolerance and encouragement have enabled me to dedicate myself fully to clinical and scientific research, resulting in a steady stream of accomplishment.

We also thank experts and colleagues, both domestically and internationally, for their guidance, assistance, and support.

MIX
Papier aus verantwortungsvollen Quellen
Paper from responsible sources
FSC® C105338

If you have any concerns about our products,
you can contact us on
ProductSafety@springernature.com

In case Publisher is established outside the EU,
the EU authorized representative is:
Springer Nature Customer Service Center GmbH
Europaplatz 3, 69115 Heidelberg, Germany

Printed by Libri Plureos GmbH
in Hamburg, Germany